Emergency
UROLOGY

David Thurtle BMec
Academic Clinical Fellow in Urology,
Cambridge University Hospitals
NHS Foundation Trust, UK

Suzanne Biers BSc MBBS MD FRCS (Urol)
Consultant Urologist,
Cambridge University Hospitals
NHS Foundation Trust, UK

Michal Sut Lek Med MMedSci FRCS (Urol)
Senior Registrar, Urology,
Cambridge University Hospitals
NHS Foundation Trust, UK

James Armitage BSc MBBS MD FRCS (Urol)
Consultant Urologist,
Cambridge University Hospitals
NHS Foundation Trust, UK

tfm Publishing Limited, Castle Hill Barns, Harley, Nr Shrewsbury, SY5 6LX, UK.
Tel: +44 (0)1952 510061; Fax: +44 (0)1952 510192
E-mail: nikki@tfmpublishing.com; Web site: www.tfmpublishing.com

First Edition: © 2017
Cover images: iStock.com (from left to right):

X-ray image of KUB, showing left kidney stone, © Sutthaburawonk
Retained Foley catheter, © ChaNaWiT
Pelvis — male false color cutaway view, © Medical Art Inc.
Kidney stones, ©John Lerskau
Background image — human kidneys anatomy, © Nerthuz

Paperback   ISBN: 978-1-910079-42-3

E-book editions: 2017
ePub   ISBN: 978-1-910079-43-0
Mobi   ISBN: 978-1-910079-44-7
Web pdf   ISBN: 978-1-910079-45-4

Printed by Gutenberg Press Ltd., Gudja Road, Tarxien, PLA 19, Malta.
Tel: +356 21897037; Fax: +356

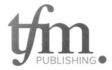

Contents

Contributing Authors

Samih Al-Hayek MD FRCS (Urol)
Consultant Urologist, Cambridge
University Hospitals NHS Foundation
Trust, UK

Tariq Ali MBBS MRCP MSc MRGP
AFHEA FRCR
Fellow in Interventional Radiology,
Cambridge University Hospitals NHS
Foundation Trust, UK

James Armitage BSc MBBS MD
FRCS (Urol)
Consultant Urologist, Cambridge
University Hospitals NHS Foundation
Trust, UK

Suzanne Biers MD FRCS (Urol)
Consultant Urologist, Cambridge
University Hospitals NHS Foundation
Trust, UK

Alexandra Colquhoun MD FRCS (Urol)
Consultant Urologist, Cambridge
University Hospitals NHS Foundation
Trust, UK

Ragada El-Damanawi MBBS MRCP
Specialist Registrar in Nephrology,
Cambridge University Hospitals NHS
Foundation Trust, UK

Andrew Fry MA MB BChir PhD FRCP
Consultant in Nephrology and Acute
Medicine, Cambridge University
Hospitals NHS Foundation Trust, UK

Tom Mitchell DPhil BMBCh FRCS (Urol)
Academic Clinical Lecturer and
Honorary Urology Registrar,
Cambridge, UK

Adam Nelson MBChB MRes MRCS AFHEA
Academic Clinical Fellow and
Honorary Urology Registrar,
Cambridge, UK

Ben Pullar MBBS FRCS (Urol)
Specialist Registrar in Urology,
Cambridge University Hospitals NHS
Foundation Trust, UK

Andrew Robb MCh FRCSEd(Paed Surg)
DipIMC(RCSEd)
Consultant Paediatric Urologist,
Birmingham Children's Hospital,
Birmingham, UK

CJ Shukla PhD FRCS (Urol)
Consultant Urologist, NHS Lothian,
Edinburgh, UK

Michal Sut Lek Med MMedSci FRCS (Urol)
Specialist Registrar, Cambridge
University Hospitals NHS Foundation
Trust, UK

Nikesh Thiruchelvam MD MBBS BSc
FRCS (Urol)
Consultant Urologist, Cambridge
University Hospitals NHS Foundation
Trust, UK

David Thurtle BMBS BMedSci MRCS
Academic Clinical Fellow in Urology,
Cambridge University Hospitals NHS
Foundation Trust, UK

Holly Weaver MA MB BCh
Foundation Doctor, Cambridge
University Hospitals NHS Foundation
Trust, UK

Andrew Winterbottom MBBCh
MRCS FRCR
Consultant Interventional Radiologist,
Cambridge University Hospitals NHS
Foundation Trust, UK

Acknowledgements

Mr Tev Aho, Consultant Urologist, Cambridge University Hospitals NHS Foundation Trust, UK: HoLEP images, Chapter 3.

Boston Scientific, Marlborough, MA, USA: AUS figures, Chapter 6.

Dr Ciaran Conway, GP Registrar, Severn Deanery, UK: hydrocoele images, Chapter 1.

Drvgaikwad. Paraphimosis image, Chapter 4. Used under Creative Commons licence 3.0. (http://creativecommons.org/licenses/by/3.0), via Wikimedia Commons.)

Elsevier Publishing Ltd, UK: Fournier's gangrene image, Chapter 4 and perineal bruising image, Chapter 5. Bullock N, Doble A, Turner W, Cuckow P. *Urology: An Illustrated Colour Text*. Elsevier, Churchill Livingstone, 2007; p 49, Fig. 3 and p138, Fig. 1.

Klemen Jagodič *et al*. Intra-operative penile fracture images, Chapter 4. Used under Creative Commons Attribution licence 2.0. Klemen Jagodič, *et al*. *Journal of Medical Case Reports* 2007; 1: 14. DOI: 10.1186/1752-1947-1-14.

Dr Abeyna Jones, Occupational Medicine Registrar and NHS Clinical Entrepreneur Fellow, King's College Hospital, UK: difficult catheterisation algorithm, Chapter 7.

Dr Olivia Kenyon, Foundation Doctor, Cambridge University Hospitals NHS Foundation Trust, UK: illustrations in Chapters 4 and 7.

Dr Jacek Libiszewski, Consultant Radiologist, Peterborough and Stamford Hospitals NHS Foundation Trust: MSCC MRI image, Chapter 6.

Mediplus Ltd, UK: images in Chapter 6 – insertion of Mediplus Ltd. S-Cath™ system and components.

Mr Joseph Norris, Academic Clinical Fellow, University College London Hospitals NHS Foundation Trust.

Mr Andrew Robb, Consultant Paediatric Urologist, Birmingham Children's Hospital: paediatric clinical images in Chapter 6.

The Resuscitation Council (UK): the ABCDE approach – Appendix 2.

The UK Sepsis Trust: Sepsis definitions and information used in Chapter 1 and Emergency Department Sepsis Screening and Action Tool – Appendix 1.

Kay Trabucchi, Urology Nurse Specialist, West Suffolk Hospital NHS Trust: bladder scan image, Chapter 3.

Dr Anne Warren, Consultant Histopathologist, Cambridge University Hospitals NHS Foundation Trust, UK: microscopy images, Chapters 2 and 3.

Dr Andrew Winterbottom, Consultant Interventional Radiologist, Cambridge University Hospitals NHS Foundation Trust: radiological figures and legends throughout the book.

Abbreviations

5-ARI	5-alpha-reductase inhibitor	β-HCG	beta-human chorionic gonadotrophin
AAA	abdominal aortic aneurysm		
ABG	arterial blood gas	CAUTI	catheter-associated urinary tract infection
Abx	antibiotics		
ACEI	angiotensin converting enzyme inhibitor	CCF	congestive cardiac failure
		CFU	colony-forming units
ACS	acute coronary syndrome	Ch	Charrière. Unit of measurement, see 'Fr'
ADH	antidiuretic hormone		
AKI	acute kidney injury	CI	contrast-induced
AML	angiomyolipoma	CIS	carcinoma in situ
ANA	antinucleic acid	CISC	clean intermittent self-catheterisation
ANCA	antineutrophil cytoplasmic antibody		
		CKD	chronic kidney disease
APTT	activated partial thromboplastin time	COPD	chronic obstructive pulmonary disease
ARB	angiotensin II receptor blocker	CPR	cardiopulmonary resuscitation
ATLS®	Advanced Trauma Life Support	CRP	C-reactive protein
ATN	acute tubular necrosis	CRT	capillary refill time
AUR	acute urinary retention	CT	computed tomography
AUS	artificial urinary sphincter	CUR	chronic urinary retention
BAUS	British Association of Urological Surgeons	CXR	chest X-ray
		DH	drug history
BCG	bacillus Calmette–Guérin	DHT	dihydrotestosterone
BD	bis in die (twice daily)	DIC	disseminated intravascular coagulopathy
BNF	British National Formulary		
BOO	bladder outlet obstruction	DMSA	dimercaptosuccinic acid scan
BP	blood pressure	DRE	digital rectal examination
BPE	benign prostatic enlargement	DSD	detrusor sphincter dyssynergia
BPH	benign prostatic hyperplasia	ECG	electrocardiography
bpm	beats/min, breaths/min	ED	erectile dysfunction
BXO	balanitis xerotica obliterans	eGFR	estimated glomerular filtration rate

ENT	ear, nose and throat	LA	local anaesthetic
EPN	emphysematous pyelonephritis	LFT	liver function test
ESR	erythrocyte sedimentation rate	LUTS	lower urinary tract symptoms
ESWL	extracorporeal shock wave lithotripsy	MAGI	male accessory gland infection
		MC&S	microscopy, culture and sensitivities
FAST	focused assessment with sonography for trauma	MRI	magnetic resonance imaging
FBC	full blood count	MSCC	metastatic spinal cord compression
FiO$_2$	fraction of inspired oxygen		
Fr	French – a measurement system for catheter diameter. 1 Fr = 1/3mm. Synonymous with Charrière, the system's French inventor	MSU	mid-stream urine
		NB	*nota bene*
		NICE	National Institute for Health and Care Excellence
		NSAIDs	non-steroidal anti-inflammatory drugs
GA	general anaesthesia		
GBM	glomerular basement membrane	NSF	nephrogenic systemic fibrosis
GFR	glomerular filtration rate	MRI	magnetic resonance imaging
GI	gastrointestinal	MRSA	methicillin-resistant *Staphylococcus aureus*
GN	glomerulonephritis		
GP	general practitioner	MRU	magnetic resonance urography
GUM	genitourinary medicine	MS	multiple sclerosis
Hb	haemoglobin	MSCC	metastatic spinal cord compression
HELLP	haemolysis, elevated liver enzymes, low platelets		
		NIV	non-invasive ventilation
HIV	human immunodeficiency virus	OD	*omni die* (once daily)
HoLEP	holmium laser enucleation of the prostate	ON	*omni nocte* (once nightly)
		PaO$_2$	partial pressure of oxygen in arterial blood
HPCUR	high-pressure chronic urinary retention		
		PCNL	percutaneous nephrolithotomy
HR	heart rate	PDE	phosphodiesterase
HSP	Henoch–Schönlein purpura	PID	pelvic inflammatory disease
IBD	inflammatory bowel disease	PMH	past medical history
ICU	intensive care unit	PO	*per os* (by mouth)
INR	International Normalised Ratio	PR	per rectum
ISC	intermittent self-catheterisation	PSA	prostate-specific antigen
ISD	intermittent self-dilatation	PTH	parathyroid hormone
ITU	intensive therapy unit	PUJ	pelviureteric junction
IV	intravenous	PV	per vagina
JVP	jugular venous pulse/pressure	PVR	post-void residual (urinary volume)
KDIGO	Kidney Disease Improving Global Outcomes		
		RCC	renal cell carcinoma
KUB	kidneys, ureters, bladder	RR	respiratory rate

SCI	spinal cord injury		TWOC	trial without catheter
SIRS	systemic inflammatory response syndrome		U&E	urea and electrolytes
SPC	suprapubic catheter		UO	urine output
STI	sexually-transmitted infection		USS	ultrasound scan
TB	tuberculosis		UTI	urinary tract infection
TDS	*ter die somendum* (three times daily)		VBG	venous blood gas
			VTE	venous thromboembolism
TIN	tubulointerstitial nephritis		VUJ	vesicoureteric junction
TRUS	transrectal ultrasound scan		VUR	vesicoureteric reflux
TUR	transurethral resection		WBC	white blood cell
TURBT	transurethral resection of bladder tumour		WCC	white cell count
			XGP	xanthogranulomatous pyelonephritis
TURP	transurethral resection of the prostate			

Preface

Urology is a specialty that often receives little attention in medical school; however, it makes up a sizeable portion of the workload in emergency departments, primary care and hospital wards.

The way urology services are delivered may increasingly mean hospitals do not have dedicated out-of-hours urology cover, such that the onus is placed on family practitioners, emergency physicians and general surgeons to manage the patient appropriately, at least initially. Emergency urology conditions can often be managed without immediate involvement of a urology specialist but require the appropriate knowledge and skills, which we aim to deliver with this new textbook.

The appeal of urology to those who chose to specialise is not only the breadth of conditions but also the ability to offer huge improvements to the quality of life for patients. Nowhere is this more true than with emergency conditions. The correct timely management of emergency problems may not only be life-saving but can also be organ-saving (i.e. in testicular torsion and upper tract trauma) and function-preserving (i.e. erectile, bladder and renal function), so averting significant future problems for a patient.

The rationale for this book was to provide a clinically-orientated practical guide and reference text for acute urological presentations for primary care physicians, junior doctors, medical students and associated health professionals from all specialties. Each clinical topic is laid out clearly with an emphasis on important information, tips and tricks, and illustrated with radiological and clinical images to highlight and concisely convey essential information. Each topic and chapter has been written by an expert on that subject.

Broadly, the book is structured 'anatomically', from the upper urinary tract down to genitoscrotal emergencies. It should be particularly relevant to junior trainees rotating through surgical specialties, primary care physicians and emergency medicine trainees; hence the content has been deliberately designed to overlap with topics in the syllabuses for these specialties.

We would like to thank all the authors for their valuable input and contributions to this *Emergency Urology* textbook, and hope our readers find this a useful and valuable tool for clinical practice.

David Thurtle
Suzanne Biers
Michal Sut
James Armitage

Chapter 1

Assessing the Unwell Urological Patient

David Thurtle and Suzanne Biers

The approach to a new urological patient should be structured and concise. This approach should include initial resuscitation if necessary, and an assessment of the urgency or severity of the patient's condition. Thereafter, a basic urological history, examination and initial investigations will help in accurately diagnosing and treating the patient.

ABCDE

Any acutely unwell or unstable patient should undergo initial rapid assessment and resuscitation using the ABCDE principles prior to formal assessment and investigation of urological problems, which can continue once the patient's condition is stable and safe. The full ABCDE approach, suggested by the Resuscitation Council, is available in Appendix 2 (pages 185–190).

HISTORY

Common urological emergency presentations include voiding difficulty or urinary retention, pain and bleeding. It is important to be able to recognise and relate symptoms to potential pathology. Obtaining a 'baseline' urological history will be useful in evaluating the current condition and will help direct long-term management.

Urinary symptoms

Lower urinary tract symptoms (LUTS) may be acute or longstanding. It is important to determine a patient's previous urinary tract function to contextualise their acute symptoms and obtain a diagnosis. LUTS are broadly categorised into storage and voiding symptoms (*Table 1.1*). Make a direct enquiry into these symptoms (see *Box 1.1* for a comprehensive tick box to follow when assessing LUTS), establish the timeframe of symptoms and any recent change.

Table 1.1 The classification of lower urinary tract symptoms.

Storage	Voiding	Infective
• Urgency	• Straining	• Frequency
• Frequency	• Incomplete bladder emptying	• Urgency
• Urinary incontinence	• Terminal dribble	• Altered urine colour or smell
• Nocturia	• Hesitancy	• Dysuria
	• Intermittent or slow stream	
	• Double-voiding	

Box 1.1 Common lower urinary tract symptoms to enquire about in a urological history.

- Daytime frequency: number of times passing urine during the day – has this changed?
- Nocturia: number of times the patient wakes at night to pass urine – has this changed?
- Hesitancy: difficulty in initiating the void, or straining to void?
- Flow: weak, strong, intermittent?
- Incomplete emptying: the sensation of not emptying the bladder completely.
- Double voiding: urinating twice in quick succession. May be a sign of incomplete bladder emptying especially if the second void volume is reasonable.
- Strangury: pain or spasm at the end or immediately after voiding.
- Urgency: unable to hold on to urine/a strong desire to go to the toilet, which is difficult to defer.
- Urgency incontinence: involuntary leak of urine if unable to reach the toilet in time (triggers can include cold weather, going from sitting to standing, key in the door lock).
- Stress urinary incontinence: urine leak with cough, sneeze or exertion.
- Dysuria: stinging or burning on passing urine.
- Haematuria: blood in the urine.
- Pneumaturia: air bubbles in the urine (specific enquiry if a patient reports recurrent UTIs and has a history of previous pelvic cancer, surgery or radiotherapy). Indicates a possible fistula between the bowel and bladder or, less commonly, infection with gas-producing bacteria.

An acute onset of storage symptoms such as urinary frequency and urgency are often caused by urinary tract infection. Be vigilant for 'red flag' symptoms that may indicate the presence of significant underlying pathology (see *Box 1.2*). Urinary incontinence is the involuntary leakage of urine. Most commonly it is reported as a chronic symptom; however, new-onset incontinence (day or night) can be related to an overflow incontinence associated with urinary retention and occasionally associated upper urinary tract obstruction

Box 1.2 Red flag-type symptoms that should alert the clinician to a possible significant pathology.

- Visible painless haematuria.
- Pelvic pain.
- Back or bone pain.
- New-onset lower limb weakness.
- Unexplained weight loss.
- Palpable pelvic mass.

and renal impairment. It is helpful to categorise the type of incontinence:

- Stress incontinence: leakage associated with raised intra-abdominal pressure such as cough.
- Urgency incontinence: associated with a strong desire to void that cannot be deferred.
- Mixed incontinence: a combination of stress and urge urinary incontinence.
- Continuous incontinence: can be caused by a urinary tract fistula such as a vesicovaginal fistula.
- Overflow incontinence: more common in men and occurs in those with chronic urinary retention.

- Nocturnal enuresis/incontinence: in males this is a significant symptom and should alert you to the possible diagnosis of high-pressure chronic retention.

Pain

A large proportion of urological presentations will be with pain. The Site, Onset, Character, Radiation, Alleviating factors, Timing, Exacerbating factors and associated Symptoms are important to establish (SOCRATES). Both loin pain and scrotal pain will often be presumed to be of urological origin, hence the focus on these below. Remember the concept of referred pain, which is commonly misleading in urological conditions (*Box 1.3*).

Box 1.3 Referred pain.

Referred pain relates to a pain felt at a distant site from the place of development. The sensation of pain from urological organs is often referred due to the embryological origin of these organs:

- Kidney pain: radiates to the back or hypochondrium.
- Ureteric pain: varies more than renal pain, and can be felt in the back, towards the abdomen or groins and in the external genitalia.
- Bladder pain: can be felt suprapubically or deeper in the pelvis. Some men report bladder pain referred to the tip of the penis with retention or infection.
- Prostate pain: often described as lower back pain, perineal, scrotal or abdominal pain; it is also sometimes described as penile tip pain.
- Penile pain: may be referred from the bladder. Pain from the penis itself is usually well localised.
- Testicular pain: pain can be referred from the distal ureters to the testes; pain originating from the testes is often felt in the lower abdomen on the ipsilateral side. If the pain is referred from the ureter, the testes are typically not tender on palpation.

This phenomenon is partly why a genital examination should be performed on male patients presenting with lower abdominal pain, and an abdominal examination performed on those with testicular pain.

Loin pain

The most common causes of acute loin pain are ureteric colic and pyelonephritis, but the differential diagnosis is wide. Ureteric colic tends to come on within seconds or minutes, coming in waves of severe pain and the patient often reports being unable to get comfortable in any position. This colicky pain is often referred to the groin or the back, or down to the genitals. The location of the pain does not necessarily correlate with the location of the stone. Sensation to the ureters is from nerves derived from spinal cord segments between T12 and L2. The same dermatome is affected (T12–L2); therefore, pain can be experienced in the back, loins, scrotum or labia majora and anterior aspects of the upper thigh. Associated symptoms of urinary urgency, frequency and strangury or referred pain to the genitals can be suggestive of a calculus in the distal ureter within the bladder wall (intramural ureter). A list of differential diagnoses for loin pain is found in Chapter 2, page 29. By far the most important differential not to miss is a leaking abdominal aortic aneurysm.

Scrotal pain

Acute scrotal pain should raise suspicion of a testicular torsion, until proven otherwise (Chapter 4, page 69). Like any ischaemic pain, this is severe and continuous. Epididymo-orchitis tends to be a less severe, dragging pain of slower onset but the history should not be relied upon alone. It is important to establish the laterality and any previous similar history of pain. Some patients may have intermittent torsion, where the testis torts and spontaneously detorts. Do not be reassured by a history of scrotal trauma, as approximately 10% of those with torsion will report recent trauma. It is unclear whether scrotal trauma is a risk factor for torsion, or whether patients retrospectively attribute blame to an otherwise innocuous injury.

History of previous urological input or intervention

Past surgical history is always important to establish. Urological procedures in the past can suggest a propensity to a certain condition, such as a previous ureteroscopy in a recurrent stone former. Anyone undergoing instrumentation of the urethra or an endoscopic procedure will be at higher risk of urethral strictures. Ask patients whether they have ever had a previous catheter insertion, and whether it was inserted with any difficulty. Any recent urological instrumentation has an associated risk of urinary tract infection.

Past medical history

It is important to establish a patient's general fitness, and to know about certain medical conditions, particularly any cause of renal impairment or propensity to disease, such as underlying malignancy, immune compromise or diabetes. A patient who has suffered from a urological condition in the past (such as stones, cystitis or epididymitis) will be at increased risk of suffering from the same disorder in the future.

Drug history

Always establish early whether a patient has any allergies. A thorough medication history will help to establish a patient's general health, clarify past medical history and provide vital information on potential interactions or contraindications to new medications. Some medications may be the cause of a patient's urinary symptoms. Pay particular attention to medications known to cause nephrotoxicity (see Chapter 2, page 19, *Box 2.2*).

EXAMINATION

Unlike some specialties, it is harder to uncover many clues to the urological diagnosis from a general examination or examination of the peripheries. Nonetheless it is important to examine the patient generally and then focus more on the area of complaint. A chaperone should always be present when performing an intimate examination. It is good practice for the presence and name of a chaperone to be recorded in the medical notes.

Systemic/general examination

Assess how unwell the patient is generally. Are they haemodynamically stable or are there any signs of systemic inflammatory response syndrome (SIRS) or sepsis (pages 12–15). Signs of cachexia, malnutrition, lethargy and pallor may be indicative of an underlying malignant process. Signs of fluid retention, altered skin pigmentation or excoriations may be suggestive of uraemia from renal failure. Gynaecomastia may be a sign of androgen deprivation therapy (used in prostate cancer) or oestrogen-producing testicular tumours (rare).

Kidneys

It is unusual for normal kidneys to be palpable. The kidneys should be examined by bimanual palpation, 'ballotting' the organ between both hands. The right is more commonly palpable as it is displaced inferiorly by the liver. A tender kidney should be obvious; percussion tenderness may also be present. Look at the skin over the flanks for any scars from previous open or percutaneous kidney operations, and any skin lesions that could be the cause of flank pain (such as shingles). Open nephrectomy may be performed via a 'rooftop' incision or a more lateral thoracolumbar incision. Laparoscopic port sites may be more difficult to see (see **Figure 1.1** for further scars from urological surgery). Auscultation in the epigastrium for renal bruits, suggestive of renal artery stenosis, may be helpful. In trauma cases, look for patterns of bruising, other significant injuries and assess for rib fracture, which is associated with an increased risk of underlying renal trauma.

Bladder

The empty bladder lies impalpable in the pelvis, posterior to the pubic symphysis. A palpable bladder is likely to have over 300ml of urine within it. The bladder may be tender in cystitis or acute retention. It is often easier to judge bladder size by percussion, with urine in the bladder dull to percussion, compared to gas-filled bowels.

A hand-held bladder scanner is a useful adjunct, though its accuracy can be variable. The most accurate assessment of bladder volume is a urinary catheter and drainage. The drained volume after catheter insertion

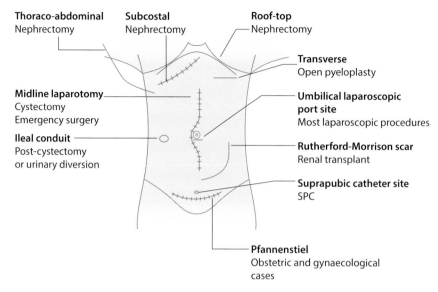

Figure 1.1 Common urological scars and the potential operation for each.

should always be recorded in the medical notes.

Prostate

Ensure the patient's verbal consent for intimate examination and arrange for a chaperone.

The prostate is traditionally examined with the patient in the left lateral position. The patient should be counselled as to what digital rectal examination (DRE) entails. The patient is placed on the edge of the couch, in the left lateral position with the knees brought up towards the chest. A gloved finger is gently inserted, with lubricant jelly, and the prostate examined. Feel the central sulcus of the prostate, and the full extent of both lobes if possible. A normal prostate is about the size of a walnut, but smooth and rubbery in consistency. Asymmetry, nodularity or a very hard gland are suspicious features of prostate cancer (**Figure 1.2**). Prostatitis tends to cause a tender, boggy prostate. A prostatic abscess may be felt as a very tender, soft lump. With benign enlargement, the prostate remains smooth and of normal consistency; the median sulcus may no longer be palpable.

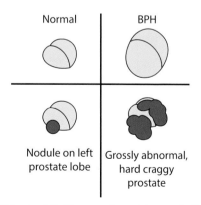

Figure 1.2 Diagram of prostate examination findings, when examined in the left lateral position. Both of the lower diagrams are likely to indicate different stages of prostate cancer.

Nuts or fruits can be used as analogies for prostate size, such as a 'walnut-sized' or 'orange-sized' gland. An accurate prostate volume can be measured using transrectal ultrasound (TRUS), or volume estimated from pelvic ultrasound.

Previous radiotherapy tends to leave a very small but palpable prostate. A high-riding prostate is a feature of trauma with urethral disruption. Absence of a palpable prostate suggests a previous prostatectomy.

Where clinically relevant, performing DRE will also give information on rectal mucosa, stool type, consistency and the presence or absence of blood on the examining finger, as well as identifying presacral masses.

Vaginal examination (where clinically relevant)

A vaginal examination is occasionally helpful in the acute urological presentation for selected cases. Ensure a chaperone is present, the patient fully understands the procedure and verbal consent has been gained. Inspect the perineum for atrophic vaginitis (seen in low oestrogen or post-menopausal women). A cough test can be used to assess for incontinence. Perform a bimanual examination to palpate for pelvic masses (in women cervical cancer can present with urinary retention). In older women, post-menopausal bleeding may suggest a gynaecological cause for new retention, so vaginal blood is an important exam finding. A Sims speculum examination can assess for prolapse.

Penis

Explain to the patient what you are going to do before examining his penis and ensure a chaperone is present. Inspect to identify conditions such as priapism (an erect and typically painful penis), penile fracture (a swollen, bruised penis), paraphimosis (a swollen prepuce or glans distal to a constricting band of skin). Retract the prepuce to inspect all of the glans, so as not to miss penile cancer. Always remember to replace the foreskin at the end of the examination. The location of the urethral meatus should be noted. Focus should be paid to any discharge from the urethral meatus: blood can be an ominous sign with trauma (indicating urethral injury); white or yellow discharge may be suggestive of a sexually-transmitted infection. In patients with urethral catheters, urethral mucus discharge may be visible around the meatus. This is washed away by antegrade urinary flow in individuals without catheters, and is a normal finding. A palpable defect can be found occasionally in penile fracture and thickened plaques can be felt in Peyronie's disease.

When describing penile abnormalities or injuries remember that in the anatomical position the penis stands erect; therefore, its ventral aspect is the underside of a flaccid penis (where the urethra lies), and the dorsal aspect is found on the upper side.

Scrotum

The scrotum is best examined when the patient is warm and relaxed. Examination should be performed both with the patient standing, when a hernia and vari-cocoele may be more obvious, and when lying supine. Whilst standing, inspect the scrotum for any skin changes or abnormalities. Assess for the presence and orientation of both testicles. The patient may be aware that one testicle lies higher than the other and can indicate if one is abnormally elevated. If there is a problem on one side, always examine the 'normal' side first, so that the difference in the abnormal side can be compared to the standard. It is useful (but not essential) to examine the patient from each side, palpating the ipsilateral testis, epididymis, cord structures and hernial orifices on that side. Assess for a cough impulse. Repeat the examination whilst lying, again examining the hernial orifices closely.

Assess for the presence of scrotal and testicular swelling. Transillumination can be used to demonstrate a hydrocoele, or large epididymal cysts in the scrotum (**Figure 1.3**). Remember that indirect genitoscrotal hernias can present with a lump in the scrotum. Testicular cancer tends to be a discrete firm mass.

Prehn's sign refers to lifting of the testicles to the level of the pubic symphysis. In the case of epididymo-orchitis the pain may be improved by performing this procedure (a 'positive Prehn's sign'). The cremasteric reflex can be elicited by lightly stroking the inner aspect of the upper thigh with a gloved hand or tongue depressor. The sensory fibres of the femoral branch of the genitofemoral nerve (L1, L2) are stimulated, synapse at the spinal cord and innervate motor fibres of the genital branch of the same nerve to cause cremasteric muscle contraction and so cause elevation of the ipsilateral testicle. This reflex is usually absent in testicular torsion.

It is important to examine the perineum, especially in the presence of infection to look for necrosis. Palpation may elicit tenderness related to prostatitis or crepitus associated with an infection with a gas-forming organism.

Groins

Inguinoscrotal pain can be caused by impingement of the ilioinguinal nerve. This can occur with inguinal hernias, or following hernia surgery. Inguinal hernias arise supero-medial to the pubic tubercle, whereas femoral hernias arise infero-lateral. Lymph nodes in the groin may suggest inflammatory or malignant conditions in the pelvis or lower limbs.

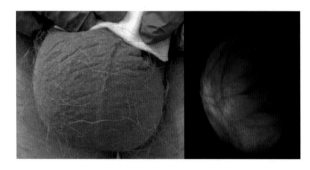

Figure 1.3 Clinical photographs demonstrating the diagnostic use of transillumination. A moderately enlarged right hemi-scrotum is shown here to transilluminate, in accordance with the underlying diagnosis of a hydrocoele. (Image courtesy of Dr C. Conway.)

Key Points

- Always examine the external genitalia of young men with acute abdominal pain, to avoid missing torsion.
- Ensure a chaperone is present, and recorded in the notes, for intimate examinations.

ROUTINE INVESTIGATIONS

Bladder scan

A bedside bladder scan provides a useful assessment of current bladder volume. In the acute setting this can help differentiate urinary retention from other abdominal pathology. These are limited by their low specificity, for example, ascitic fluid may be misinterpreted by the device as bladder contents.

Flow analysis

A urinary flowmeter (**Figure 1.4**) is useful in the outpatient setting to assess patterns of bladder emptying.

Urinalysis

Dipstick urinalysis (**Figure 1.5**) is the simplest of procedures yet can yield large amounts of information. A mid-stream sample is best, but any sample can be a useful screening tool. Watch for false positives in the context of visible haematuria, which may lead to all parameters appearing positive. If any suspicion of infection exists, a sample should be sent to microbiology. *Table 1.2* explains the significance of each parameter. (See also *Table 3.5* in Chapter 3).

Urinary or serum beta-human chorionic gonadotrophin (β-HCG)

β-HCG is elevated in pregnancy. It must be checked in all women of potential childbearing age in the context of abdominal pain and before any irradiating imaging.

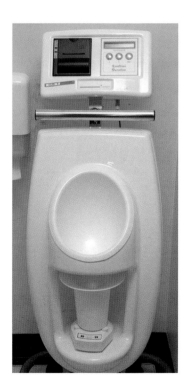

Figure 1.4 Urinary flowmeter.

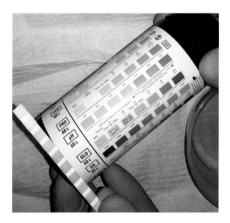

Figure 1.5 Dipstick urinalysis. Automated point-of-care urinalysis machines are now widely used.

Table 1.2 Common dipstick urinalysis results and their significance.

Specific gravity	A measure of the amount of solute in the urine compared to the amount in water (1.00). Decreased (<1.005) may indicate excessive fluid intake, or an inability to concentrate urine (acute tubular necrosis, glomerulonephritis, diabetes insipidus). Increased (>1.035) suggests concentrated urine, which may be due to dehydration, or artificially elevated by urine contamination, proteinuria or glycosuria.
pH	Kidneys usually maintain the acidity of urine at between pH 5.5–6.5. Low urinary pH (acidic urine) may reflect systemic acidosis, or be artificially low because of dietary or medicinal causes such as cranberries or methenamine hippurate (Hiprex). High urinary pH (alkaline urine) may reflect systemic alkalosis; some urinary tract infections can cause alkalinisation due to bacterial effects on urea; and drugs and medications can alkalinise urine (e.g. sodium bicarbonate).
Protein	Dipstick urinalysis is most sensitive for albumin. Anything above 'trace' may be significant and may reflect primary renal disorders (e.g. nephrotic syndrome) or cardiovascular causes (e.g. congestive cardiac failure), as well as functional polyuria of various causes (e.g. pregnancy) or as a result of certain medications. Any doubt should lead to a 24-hour urinary protein collection, where >150mg/24h is abnormal.
Leukocytes	Leukocyte esterase activity acts as a surrogate for the presence of white cells (leukocytes). This correlates with bacteriuria in about 80%; however, false positives are common with contaminated samples, and false negatives may occur with concurrent antibiotics.
Nitrites	Most Gram-negative bacteria (e.g. *E. coli*) will convert nitrates to nitrites, such that nitrites are a surrogate for bacteriuria. However, some bacteria, including most enterococci, will not produce nitrites, so sensitivity is about 80%.
Blood	Haemolysed and non-haemolysed blood can be detected. There are a wide range of potential causes (*Box 3.2*, page 53) including infection, calculi, trauma and urological malignancy. A 'trace' result is considered normal, and 1+ or more is a positive finding.
Bilirubin	Bilirubin should not be present in the urine of normal individuals. It reflects the presence of a conjugated bilirubinaemia, seen in hepatobiliary disease. Note that urobilinogen is not abnormal when found in the urine at low concentrations.
Glucose	Glycosuria usually reflects hyperglycaemia (e.g. diabetes mellitus) or insufficiency of glucose resorption in the kidneys (e.g. renal tubular acidosis or pregnancy). Serum glucose and urinary or plasma ketones should be measured.
Ketones	Ketones are the result of incomplete fat metabolism. Ketonuria may reflect low carbohydrate diets, starvation or ketosis associated with diabetes.

FAST scan (focused assessment with sonography for trauma)

Developed in the context of trauma, 'FAST' scans use ultrasound and have become far more available. Most senior emergency physicians are trained in their use. This rapid bedside examination adjunct can give useful information on gross intra-abdominal abnormalities. Abdominal aortic aneurysms can be assessed quickly. In trained hands, these machines can also be useful to assess for gross hydronephrosis and bladder distension.

Blood tests

- Blood gas: a useful way of getting quick results, especially haemoglobin, potassium, lactate and pH.
- Urea and electrolytes: for baseline or acute renal impairment.
- Coagulation screen: vital when considering surgical or radiological intervention, or in the context of active bleeding.
- Full blood count: assess for neutrophilia and haemoglobin level. A low platelet count can be an early sign of sepsis and is important when considering surgery.
- C-reactive protein (CRP): a non-specific marker of infection/inflammation. This is useful to monitor clinical progress or response to treatment.
- Calcium and uric acid levels: if elevated can be causative for stone disease. Hypercalcaemia can cause acute pain in its own right. If raised serum calcium is identified, remember to check parathyroid hormone (PTH) levels also (to look for hyperparathyroidism).
- Prostate-specific antigen (PSA): although serum PSA levels will be raised with infection, or prostatitis, it is usually not helpful in the acute

setting unless a patient presents with manifestations of advanced prostate cancer. PSA should be used only after careful counselling of patients about the potential sequelae of an abnormal result. Some evidence suggests PSA can take 6 months to return to baseline levels after an infection, although most would accept the result to be accurate after waiting 4 weeks after a treated urinary tract infection (UTI) or instrumentation.

- Blood cultures: should be performed in all patients with suspected systemic infection, prior to antibiotic delivery.

IMAGING INVESTIGATIONS

Computed tomography (CT)

CT of the kidneys, ureters and bladder (CTKUB) is a non-contrast CT scan of the abdomen. CTKUB is the gold standard investigation for renal or ureteric colic. It may also help rule out or determine other causes for pain such as abdominal aortic aneurysm. CT (with intravenous [IV] contrast) is the gold standard in trauma if indications are met (*Box 5.2*, page 94).

Ultrasound scan (USS)

Ultrasound avoids the use of radiation and provides rapid information. However, it is heavily user-dependent and is less useful in patients with larger body habitus.

USS KUB is used in UTI/pyelonephritis to exclude an obstructed system and used in potential stone disease when the radiation of CT is contraindicated, although it is generally not good at detecting ureteric stones. In acute kidney injury it can suggest or exclude an obstructive cause.

USS is useful in the investigation of patients with an acute scrotum and for follow-up of testicular problems such as epididymo-orchitis.

Urethrogram/cystogram

Dynamic fluoroscopy screening of the urethra (urethrogram) or bladder (cystogram) with injection of contrast via a Foley catheter are useful where concerns exist regarding trauma to the bladder or urethra or both, either at the acute event, or for follow-up to ensure resolution. Ensure that an adequate volume of contrast (300ml) is used for the cystogram study. Oblique views are helpful and a repeated image after bladder emptying is important as it may reveal a urine leak initially concealed by a bladder distended with contrast.

Magnetic resonance imaging (MRI)

Emergency MRI of the spine is necessary when there are concerns of malignant spinal cord compression with neurological symptoms, even out of hours.

- MRI of the prostate and bladder are used in oncological staging of these cancers.
- MRI can also be useful to assess prostatic abscesses.
- MRI is occasionally useful in cases of penile fracture and priapism, but in this setting its use is generally restricted to specialist centres.

SEPSIS

Sepsis is defined as the presence of systemic inflammatory response syndrome (SIRS) in the context of a suspected or confirmed infection. Patients can become very unstable, very quickly; it is a time-critical condition. Immediate management should be instigated within 1 hour. SIRS requires only two of the criteria listed in *Box 1.4*. The high mortality rates of sepsis, severe sepsis and septic shock are demonstrated in *Table 1.3*.

Urinary sepsis or 'urosepsis' is a specific subdivision of sepsis; it requires the same parameters as sepsis and a proven pathogen on urine microbiology. The term is often used inappropriately to describe patients with simple UTIs, or used before a positive urinary culture has been acquired. However, suspected sepsis should be taken seriously and patients assessed quickly.

Urinary sepsis can be anticipated in some patient groups such as those with the presence of, or manipulation of, an

Box 1.4 Systemic inflammatory response syndrome definition (≥2 of the following):

- Temperature: >38.3°C or <36.0°C.
- Heart rate: >90 bpm.
- Respiratory rate: >20 bpm (or $PaCO_2$<4.3kPa).
- White cell count: >12 ×10^9/L or <4 ×10^9/L.
- Blood glucose: >7.7mmol/L in the absence of diabetes.
- New confusion/drowsiness.

Table 1.3 Mortality for septic patients.

Severity	Definition	Group mortality
Uncomplicated sepsis	SIRS + presumed or confirmed infection	10%
Severe sepsis	Sepsis + one or more organ dysfunction criteria (other than shock) *	35%
Septic shock	Sepsis + shock **	50%

*Organ dysfunction criteria:
– Bilateral lung infiltrates + new need for oxygen to maintain saturations >90%, OR
– Bilateral lung infiltrates with PaO_2/FiO_2 ratio <300mmHg or 39.9kPa.
– Lactate >2.0mmol/L.
– Serum creatinine >176.8µmol/L OR
– Urine output <0.5ml/kg/h for 2 successive hours.
– INR >1.5 or APTT >60s.
– Platelet count <100 × 10^9/L.
– Bilirubin >34.2µmol/L.

**Shock criteria:
– Lactate >4mmol/L at any time point.
– Hypotension persisting after 30ml/kg IV fluid, defined as systolic blood pressure <90mmHg, mean blood pressure <65mmHg, or a fall >40mmHg from the patient's usual systolic blood pressure.

(Table 1.3, Box 1.4 and Box 1.5 reproduced with the kind permission of the UK Sepsis Trust. http://sepsistrust.org).

indwelling urinary catheter (urethral, suprapubic, or nephrostomy), those undergoing urological surgery or those with urinary tract obstruction. Some patient groups are at higher risk of sepsis such as those with diabetes, intensive care patients, and the immunocompromised.

Management
Good management of sepsis relies on three principles: early recognition, urgent intervention and timely escalation. In reality, the assessment of the septic patient should combine investigation, with initial resuscitation and treatment.

An example protocol for the initial management of suspected sepsis from the UK Sepsis Trust is available in Appendix 1.

Early recognition
A high suspicion of sepsis should persist for hospital inpatients. All emergency depart-

ment and ward staff should be trained in the early recognition of potentially septic patients. A full set of observations must be performed and a serum lactate should be measured urgently.

Early recognition should be coupled with risk stratification. The serum lactate level is a good indicator of severity; an initial lactate ≥4 correlates with a 28-day mortality of over 25%. The severity of sepsis should be established early; a stand-alone term of 'sepsis' is too broad, and not acceptable. Septic shock warrants immediate escalation.

Urgent intervention

Recent sepsis campaigns have focused on initial goal-directed therapy. The initial 'Sepsis Six' (*Box 1.5*) should be implemented within 1 hour of identification or a suspicion of sepsis and confirmation of diagnosis should not be awaited. Antibiotic choice should be driven by the likely source, previous culture results and local antibiotic-prescribing guidelines. Most sepsis guidelines suggest initial broad-spectrum antibiotics. UK guidelines suggest up to 30ml/kg of crystalloid fluid should be quickly delivered in divided doses to those with evidence of hypoperfusion.

After initial resuscitation, the focus shifts to source control. In urinary sepsis this may mean catheterisation of a full bladder or decompression of an infected obstructed kidney (see Chapter 2). Alternative sources of sepsis should be considered when the cause is unclear; a full 'septic screen' (*Box 1.6*) should be considered if doubt persists.

Box 1.5 'The Sepsis Six'.

1. Administer high-flow oxygen.
2. Take blood cultures and consider an infective source.
3. Administer IV antibiotics.
4. Give IV fluid resuscitation.
5. Check haemoglobin and serial lactates.
6. Commence hourly urine output measurement.

Box 1.6 The 'septic screen'.

Potential infective source and investigation

- Urinary: urinalysis, microscopy, culture and sensitivity.
- Respiratory: chest X-ray (CXR), sputum culture.
- Neurological: lumbar puncture.
- Skin: expose and examine +/- swab.
- Ear, nose, throat: examine throat and ears (especially important in children).
- Gastrointestinal: stool cultures, erect CXR, CT abdomen.
- Blood-borne infection: blood culture.
- Line infection: blood culture from line.

Timely escalation

It is vital the right individuals and teams are involved early in the care of patients with sepsis. The UK Sepsis Trust recommends all patients with septic shock or severe sepsis are reviewed by a senior clinician (registrar grade or above) within 60 minutes of diagnosis. Septic shock may require vasopressor or inotropic support, which will require a critical care bed. Early involvement of the critical care outreach team, or a similar resource is vital.

Key Points

- Have a high index of suspicion for sepsis in any unwell patient.
- Intervene and involve senior clinicians early.

Chapter 2

Upper Urinary Tract Emergencies

Ragada El-Damanawi and Andrew Fry[1] / Ben Pullar and Samih Al-Hayek[2,3]

ACUTE KIDNEY INJURY[1]

Definition and staging

Acute kidney injury (AKI) is defined as a rapid decline in glomerular filtration rate that occurs over hours to days. It results in the accumulation of nitrogenous waste products including urea and creatinine, plus reduced urine output.

The 2012 KDIGO (Kidney Disease Improving Global Outcomes) definition is one of the most recognised (*Box 2.1*) and classifies AKI into three stages based on severity (*Table 2.1*).

Epidemiology

It is now recognised that even a modest acute reduction in kidney function is associated with an increased risk of in-hospital mortality. There is also an increased risk of developing chronic kidney disease (CKD) and cardiovascular disease in the longer term. About 5-10% of general hospital admissions and 50% of all Intensive therapy unit (ITU) admissions have AKI. In those with AKI requiring renal replacement therapy, the overall mortality remains high at >50%.

Box 2.1 KDIGO AKI definition.

AKI is defined as any of the following (not graded):

- Increase in serum creatinine by ≥0.3mg/dL (≥26.5µmol/L) within 48 hours.

OR

- Increase in serum creatinine to ≥1.5 × baseline, which is known or presumed to have occurred within the prior 7 days

OR

- Urine volume <0.5ml/kg/h for 6 hours.

Causes and classification

The causes of AKI can be classified into pre-renal, intrinsic renal and post-renal.

Pre-renal AKI

Pre-renal AKI is caused by renal hypoperfusion. It is related to loss of blood volume and/or blood pressure (BP). There is no injury to the renal parenchyma, and restoration of renal blood flow restores glomerular filtration, reversing AKI (**Figure 2.1**).

Table 2.1 Stages of AKI.

Stage	Serum creatinine	Urine output
1	1.5–1.9 × baseline OR ≥0.3mg/dL (≥26.5µmol/L) increase	<0.5ml/kg/h for 6–12h
2	2.0–2.9 × baseline	<0.5ml/kg/h for ≥12h
3	3.0 × baseline OR Increase in serum creatinine to ≥4.0mg/dL (≥353.6µmol/L) OR Initiation of renal replacement therapy OR Decrease in eGFR to <35ml/min per 1.73m^2 (in those <18 years old)	<0.3ml/kg/h for ≥24h OR Anuria for ≥12h

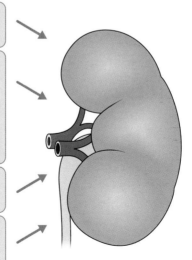

Reduced cardiac output
- Heart failure: ischaemia, arrhythmias, pericardial disease

Reduced effective circulatory blood volume
- Renal diuretics
- Gastrointestinal: diarrhoea and vomiting
- Third space losses, e.g. pancreatitis
- Skin, e.g. burns
- Cirrhosis

Reduced blood pressure
- Vasodilation: septic shock and anaphylaxis

Vasomotor changes
- ACEIs: dilatation of efferent arteriole
- NSAIDs: constriction of afferent arteriole

Figure 2.1 Causes of pre-renal acute kidney injury.

Intrinsic AKI

Intrinsic renal AKI refers to conditions that affect the glomeruli, tubules, interstitium or the vasculature of the kidneys. The commonest causes include sepsis, nephrotoxins *(Box 2.2)* and ischaemia (**Figure 2.2**).

Acute tubular necrosis

Just under half (about 45%) of all cases of AKI are due to acute tubular necrosis (ATN). The two major causes of ATN are ischaemia and nephrotoxins. ATN represents the endpoint of pre-renal AKI. In ATN, a prolonged insult leads to parenchymal damage, and the resulting AKI does not promptly resolve on restoration of glomerular filtration.

Contrast-induced AKI (CI-AKI)

This is defined as AKI within 72 hours of receiving iodinated contrast. It occurs in 1–2% of adults with normal renal function who receive contrast and it usually resolves within 5 days, although some individuals

Box 2.2 Nephrotoxic medications listed by mechanism of nephrotoxicity.

1. **Pre-renal (low BP or volume depletion)**
   Antihypertensives, diuretics

2. **Renal vasoconstriction**
   NSAIDs, ACEIs, ARBs, radio-contrast agents, cyclosporin, tacrolimus

3. **Glomerulonephritis**
   D-penicillamine, hydralazine, propylthiouracil

4. **Acute tubular necrosis**
   Amphotericin, aminoglycosides, tenofovir, cidofovir, cisplatin, heavy metals

5. **Acute interstitial nephritis**
   Antibiotics (penicillin, rifampicin, cephalosporin, ciprofloxacin), NSAIDs, proton pump inhibitors, diuretics

6. **Obstruction**
   Crystal formation: aciclovir, methotrexate, ethylene glycol

   Urinary retention: anticholinergics, tricyclic antidepressants

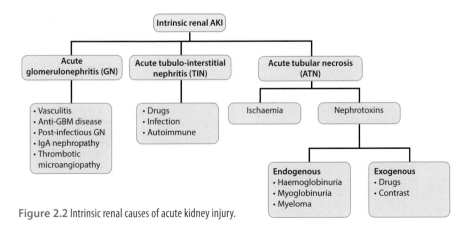

Figure 2.2 Intrinsic renal causes of acute kidney injury.

are at increased risk (*Table 2.2*). There are two main mechanisms: 1) the contrast is vasoactive causing significant afferent arteriolar vasoconstriction and therefore a reduction in blood flow to the glomerulus; 2) it is directly toxic to the tubules.

In high-risk patients it should be considered whether a contrast-enhanced scan is necessary or alternative imaging would be sufficient. *Table 2.3* outlines other measures to prevent CI-AKI. The use of magnetic resonance imaging (MRI) with gadolinium contrast should also be avoided in those with a low estimated glomerular filtration rate (eGFR) (<30ml/min) due to its association with nephrogenic systemic fibrosis (NSF) – a rare condition where there is severe fibrosis of the skin and deeper structures (with significant morbidity and mortality).

Table 2.4 outlines the distinguishing features of pre-renal and intrinsic renal AKI (including established acute tubular necrosis [ATN] as intrinsic). If in doubt, or if AKI persists, a renal biopsy is often diagnostic and helpful in excluding other treatable causes.

Post-renal AKI

Post-renal AKI is caused by obstruction of the urinary tract and may be categorised as either supra-vesical or infra-vesical, depending upon the level of obstruction in relation to the bladder (**Figure 2.3**).

Table 2.2 Risk factors for CI-AKI.

CKD with eGFR <60ml/min
Age >75 years
Diabetes
Heart failure
Hypovolaemia
Concurrent nephrotoxins: NSAIDs, aminoglycosides
Contrast: large volumes and intra-arterial administration

CI-AKI: contrast-induced acute kidney injury; CKD: chronic kidney disease; eGFR: estimated glomerular filtration rate; NSAID: non-steroidal anti-inflammatory drug.

Table 2.3 Measures to prevent CI-AKI.

Consider alternative imaging
Stop nephrotoxins (NSAIDs, ACEI, ARB)
Pre-hydration with normal saline
Reduce volume of contrast
Low or iso-osmolar contrast
Measure renal function 24–48h post-contrast

ACEI: angiotensin converting enzyme inhibitor; ARB: angiotensin receptor II blocker; CI-AKI: contrast-induced acute kidney injury; NSAID: non-steroidal anti-inflammatory drug.

Table 2.4 Distinguishing features of pre-renal and intrinsic renal AKI.

	Pre-renal AKI	Intrinsic renal AKI
BP	Hypotension common	Normal or elevated
Volume status (jugular venous pressure, postural BP)	Evidence of hypovolaemia	Normal
Urine dipstick	Unremarkable	Blood and protein (more in glomerulonephritis than ATN and acute interstitial nephritis)
Urine microscopy	Unremarkable	Red cell casts pathognomonic of acute glomerulonephritis
Response to effective fluid challenge	Improvement in urine output	No effect

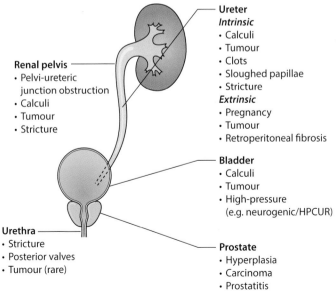

Figure 2.3 Post-renal causes of acute kidney injury.

Presentation

Table 2.5 outlines the main clinical presentation of AKI. It is most frequently encountered in the setting of another acute illness.

A careful history is often key to determining the underlying cause of AKI. Ask about recent illnesses, changes in medication (including over-the-counter drugs), previous renal history (is this new AKI or known CKD?).

Table 2.5 Clinical features of AKI.

Non-specifically unwell
Reduced urine output
Disordered volume status: Fluid overloaded Dehydration
Hyperkalaemia: cardiac arrest or arrhythmias
Uraemia: Skin: dry skin, pruritis, uraemic frosting (last sign) GI: nausea, anorexia, weight loss Nervous system: involuntary movement (restless legs), peripheral and autonomic neuropathy, psychological disturbances, encephalopathy Haematological: anaemia, bleeding
Sexual dysfunction and reduced fertility

GI: gastrointestinal.

Investigation

A simple urine dipstick is very important. Pre-renal and post-renal causes generally produce an unremarkable urine dipstick result. An 'active' urine dip (blood and protein) could indicate an intrinsic cause such as a glomerulonephritis.

Look for and treat life-threatening complications first such as abnormalities identified on electrocardiography (ECG) or hyperkalaemia identified on urea and electrolytes (U&E) and then consider other blood tests (*Table 2.6*). Imaging in the form of a basic urinary tract ultrasound scan can help to rule out obstruction. Finally, once pre- and post-renal causes have been excluded, a renal biopsy is helpful in differentiating the varying causes of intrinsic renal disease, especially in the presence of an 'active' urine dip. It is vital to determine the underlying cause of AKI as this directs the treatment and offers the best chance of reversal.

Management

In pre-renal AKI it is important to achieve and maintain haemodynamic stability. Fluid resuscitation is key and dependent on accurate clinical assessment of fluid balance. Crystalloids should be given, except in the case of bleeding, where blood and blood products are indicated (*Table 2.7*).

The management of AKI can be divided into general supportive measures (*Table 2.8*) and renal replacement therapy. The indications for renal replacement therapy are outlined in *Table 2.9*. In particular, obstruction should always be excluded, especially in oliguric and anuric patients with no other obvious cause (e.g. no overt haemodynamic disturbance).

Table 2.6 Key investigations in AKI.

Urine dip Evidence of infection, or intrinsic renal disease
Blood tests FBC: • Anaemia: haemolysis or active bleed • WCC: raised in sepsis • ESR: raised in SLE, myeloma U&E: • Increased plasma urea: creatinine ratio more likely pre-renal cause • Increased plasma creatinine: urea ratio makes obstruction and intrinsic disease more likely • Hyperkalaemia: associated with life-threatening arrhythmias LFT: • Abnormal in hepatorenal syndrome Calcium: • Hypercalcaemia is seen with malignancy and myeloma Creatine kinase: • Rhabdomyolysis: consider in patients with a history of burns, crush injuries or lying for a prolonged time Immunology screen: • ANA: positive in autoimmune disease • ANCA: small vessel vasculitis: • Cytoplasmic ANCA – PR3 antigen – granulomatosis with polyangiitis • Perinuclear ANCA – MPO antigen – microscopic polyangiitis and Churg Strauss syndrome* • Anti-GBM: Goodpasture's disease** – an important cause of pulmonary–renal syndrome • Myeloma screen: serum free light chains, protein and urine electrophoresis
Imaging: • Ultrasound renal tract (urgent) • Exclude obstruction • Ensure presence of 2 kidneys and assess size: small scarred kidneys suggest CKD
Renal biopsy: • Mainly to identify intrinsic renal disease

*Churg Strauss syndrome, also known as eosinophilic granulomatosis with polyangiitis, is a disorder characterised by inflammation of the small to medium sized blood vessels (vasculitis). Its features include adult-onset asthma, peripheral blood eosinophilia and vasculitis affecting the lungs, heart, kidney, nerves and skin.
**Goodpasture's disease is an autoimmune condition where antiglomerular basement membrane (anti-GBM) antibodies attack the basement membrane structure within the kidneys and alveoli causing an acute glomerulonephritis and lung haemorrhage. It makes up an important cause of pulmonary–renal syndrome.

ANA: antinucleic acid; ANCA: antineutrophil cytoplasmic antibody; CKD: chronic kidney disease; ESR: erythrocyte sedimentation rate; FBC: full blood count; LFT: liver function test; SLE: systemic lupus erythematosus; U&E: urea and electrolytes; WCC: white cell count.

Table 2.7 Fluid resuscitation in pre-renal AKI.

Assess fluid balance:
- Pulse: tachycardia - BP: hypertension or hypotension - Jugular venous pressure - Evidence of pulmonary oedema - Urine output
Management:
- Give 500ml crystalloid fluid bolus (reduce to 250ml in those with cardiac failure or >75 years old) - Reassess fluid balance - If required give further 500ml of crystalloid (250ml in those with cardiac failure or >75 years old) - Continue maintenance fluids until euvolaemic - If the patient remains oligoanuric despite adequate filling, defined as having volume unresponsive AKI, they require input from a nephrologist

BP: blood pressure.

Table 2.8 General supportive management.

Investigate and treat the underlying cause
Achieve normal haemodynamic status – fluids, vasopressor or inotropic support
Adjust dose and frequency of medications appropriately for level of renal function – renal drug handbook or pharmacist may help
Avoid nephrotoxins – ACEI, NSAID, aminoglycosides (*Box 2.2*)
Avoid hyperglycaemia
Nutritional support

ACEI: angiotensin converting enzyme inhibitor; NSAID: non-steroidal anti-inflammatory drug.

Table 2.9 Indications for renal replacement therapy.

Resistant hyperkalaemia
Acid–base disturbances – metabolic acidosis
Volume overload/pulmonary oedema refractory to diuretics
Severe uraemia causing encephalopathy, pericarditis, coagulopathy

The indications for referral to a nephrologist are outlined in *Table 2.10*. If the cause of AKI is clear, e.g. obstruction or dehydration, and responds to management with rapid improvement, nephrology input is generally not required. Patients who are haemodynamically unstable, or those with multi-organ failure are better managed in an intensive care setting.

It is important to acknowledge that renal replacement therapy may not be appropriate for all patients with the indications above, for example, patients with metastatic cancer with a poor prognosis.

Hyperkalaemia

Hyperkalaemia can result in life-threatening arrhythmias and cardiac arrest. It is therefore important to monitor the patient for ECG changes (**Figure 2.4**) and treat hyperkalaemia promptly (*Table 2.11*).

Table 2.10 Indications for referral to a nephrologist.

Patients meeting the criteria for renal replacement therapy
Diagnosis requires specialist input, e.g. vasculitis, GN or TIN
Cause of AKI unclear
Inadequate response to initial treatment
Renal transplant patient
Stage 3 AKI
Pre-existing advanced CKD (CKD 4 and 5)

AKI: acute kidney injury; CKD: chronic kidney disease; GN: glomerulonephritis; TIN: tubulointerstitial nephritis.

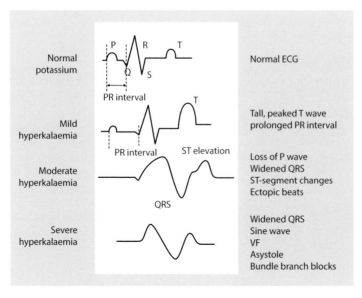

Figure 2.4 Electrocardiography changes associated with hyperkalaemia.

Table 2.11 Treatment of hyperkalaemia.

1) Stabilise the myocardium
10ml of 10% calcium gluconate IV over 2 min (remember this does not affect the potassium level)
2) Measures to reduce serum potassium **(move potassium from extracellular to intracellular compartments)**

Low potassium diet:
  • Patients should avoid potassium-rich foods including almonds, dried fruit,
    bananas, chocolate and baked potatoes
 	
Insulin–dextrose:
  • 10 units of Actrapid® in 50ml of 50% dextrose over 20 min. Potassium will
    decrease within 15 minutes. Glucose levels should be monitored carefully to
    avoid hypoglycaemia
 	
Beta 2 agonists:
  • 10–20mg of nebulised salbutamol. Be careful as can cause tachycardia and
    precipitate arrhythmia
 	
Isotonic (1.26%) sodium bicarbonate:
  • Use under expert guidance only

3) Remove potassium from the body

Cation exchange resins:
  • Calcium resonium or sodium polystyrene sulphonate. Removes potassium
    from the blood in the gut in exchange for sodium. Works slowly, over hours.
    Ideally avoid as these drugs can cause constipation, colonic ulceration and
    necrosis
 	
Dialysis:
  • If the above measures fail, treatment-resistant hyperkalaemia is an
    indication for haemodialysis or haemofiltration

RENAL COLIC[2]

Background

Patients presenting with acute loin pain with suspected renal colic represent a significant proportion of the acute presentations to urologists. The priority when assessing a patient with suspected renal colic is to exclude other life-threatening causes of pain such as a leaking abdominal aortic aneurysm (AAA). It is also important to identify an infected and obstructed kidney (pyonephrosis), which may require urgent decompression (either with a ureteric stent or a nephrostomy).

Epidemiology

The prevalence of stone disease is increasing across the developed world. This appears to be due to both an increased incidence in stones and increased detection of asymptomatic renal stones on imaging. It is estimated that the lifetime risk for formation of renal stones is 12% for men and 7% for women. Approximately 70% of renal calculi present in patients between the ages of 20 and 50 years. Once a patient has had one kidney stone the probability of a future stone episode is dramatically increased. It is estimated that up to 10% of men with a calcium oxalate stone will have a further stone within 1 year, and up to 50% will have further stone episodes within 10 years.

Causes

The causes of stone formation are often multifactorial and include both patient and environmental factors (*Box 2.3*). The most important factor that predisposes to stone formation (and which may be easily addressed) is low fluid intake (<1.5L per day). Young patients and recurrent stone

Box 2.3 Risk factors for stone formation.

Patient factors

- Age: peak incidence age 20–50 years.
- Sex: more common in males.
- Positive family history.
- Personal history of renal stones.
- Inflammatory bowel disease.

Modifiable risk factors

- Low fluid intake.
- Diet (especially high intake of animal protein).

formers require more specialist metabolic investigation. The acute pain is often due to an obstructing calculus at one of the narrowest parts of the ureter. **Figure 2.5** shows the positions where stones most commonly become impacted and cause obstruction:

- Pelviureteric junction (PUJ).
- Ureteric narrowing as the ureters cross the iliac vessels at the level of the pelvic brim.
- Vesicoureteric junction (VUJ), which is usually the narrowest of these.

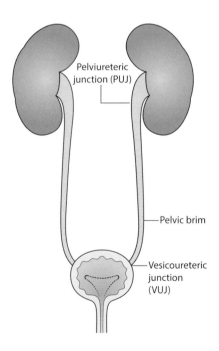

Figure 2.5 The locations at which stones most commonly obstruct the ureter.

Presentation

Patients with ureteric stones often present with acute 'renal colic' – sudden onset, severe unilateral loin to groin pain that is colicky in nature. It is often more accurate to use the term 'ureteric colic' rather than 'renal colic' as it tends to be the ureteric passage of stones that is painful. However, the two terms are often used interchangeably. Stones in the kidney are often asymptomatic and may therefore be detected as an incidental finding during the investigation of other symptoms. They may, however, present with haematuria or urinary tract infection (UTI).

In the acute setting, other urological and non-urological causes of acute loin pain should be considered, especially the possibility of a ruptured AAA in an elderly patient with no history of previous renal stone disease (*Box 2.4*).

Symptoms

- Acute severe colicky loin pain (with or without radiation to the ipsilateral groin and testicle or labia – classical renal colic).
- Usually the patient cannot find a comfortable position.
- Nausea and vomiting are common.
- The patient may report visible haematuria.
- If the stone is causing obstruction, the patient may get symptoms of AKI or even be anuric (which should raise suspicion of an obstructing stone in a single functioning kidney or bilateral obstructing ureteric stones).
- Fever or rigors are important indicators of possible associated infection (obstructed infected kidney).

Box 2.4 Differential diagnosis of acute loin pain.

Urological causes

- Obstruction: may be due to a stone, clot (e.g. **Figure 2.6**), ureteric tumour, PUJ obstruction.
- Infection: UTI/pyelonephritis.

Non-urological causes

- Leaking abdominal aortic aneurysm (the most important diagnosis to exclude in the acute setting).
- Surgical causes: appendicitis (especially if retrocaecal), inflammatory bowel disease, diverticulitis, bowel obstruction, etc.
- Gynaecological causes: ectopic pregnancy, pelvic inflammatory disease, ovarian pathology (e.g. torted ovarian cyst).
- Medical: pneumonia, myocardial infarction.

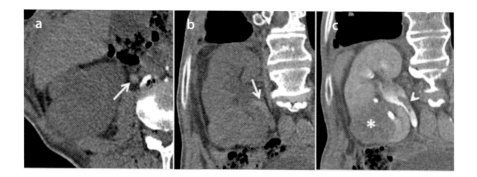

Figure 2.6 Clot colic. Non-contrast axial (**a**) and coronal (**b**) with delayed phase coronal (**c**) CT images of the right kidney showing a high-density clot in the proximal ureter (arrow image **a** and **b**), seen as a filling defect (arrow head image **c**) causing mild hydronephrosis due to the lower pole renal cell carcinoma (asterisk).

Examination

- Routine observations (temperature, heart rate [HR], respiratory rate [RR], BP and urine output [UO]).
- Abdominal and loin examination mainly to exclude other causes of pain (e.g. ruptured AAA, appendicitis).
- External genitalia to exclude alternative diagnoses such as testicular torsion.
- Features of AKI/uraemia (e.g. nausea, vomiting, fatigue, muscle cramps, pruritus, mental state changes, visual changes, thirst).

Investigation

- Urine analysis +/- urine culture (dipstick haematuria is present in approximately 80% of patients with stones but decreases as time passes).
- Pregnancy test (if applicable).
- Bloods: FBC, U&E, C-reactive protein (CRP), clotting screen (in case an invasive procedure is necessary), blood culture if there is fever.
- Basic metabolic screen if a stone is present: calcium, uric acid.
- Blood glucose (+/- HbA1c if poorly controlled diabetes is suspected).
- Stone for analysis (if passed/extracted to help with potential strategies for prevention). The most common stone types are demonstrated in *Box 2.5*.
- Urgent imaging: most departments regard non-contrast computed tomography of the kidneys, ureters, bladder (CT KUB) as first line as it has a high sensitivity and can detect other causes of abdominal pain. A plain abdominal (KUB) X-ray, if a stone was confirmed on CT, is useful in the follow-up of radio-opaque stones. In children

or pregnant women, ultrasound is the initial imaging of choice to look for hydronephrosis and the presence of stones.

Box 2.5 Types of stone.

- Calcium oxalate (70–80%).
- Uric acid (10%).
- Calcium phosphate and calcium oxalate (10%).
- Struvite: infection stones (2–20%).
- Cystine (1%).
- Pure calcium phosphate: rare.
- Others: drug, xanthine: rare.

Treatment

Acute renal colic is extremely painful and often assessment is difficult until adequate analgesia has been administered, a priority in the management of such patients. Non-steroidal anti-inflammatory drugs (NSAIDs, e.g. diclofenac 100mg per rectum) offer excellent analgesia where there are no contraindications to their use. Opioids with antiemetics are an alternative if NSAIDs cannot be used.

Treatment will be tailored to the individual patient and will depend upon both patient and stone factors. *Box 2.6* outlines some specific indications for urgent decompression of a kidney with an obstructing calculus. Three clinical scenarios follow below: a small ureteric stone, an obstructing stone with sepsis and a staghorn calculi.

Box 2.6 Indications for ureteric stent/nephrostomy insertion in a patient with a ureteric stone.

- Unremitting pain.
- AKI.
- Stone in a single kidney (or functionally single kidney).
- Sepsis.
- Bilateral obstruction or extravasation of urine.
- Stone size (and therefore unlikely to pass spontaneously; this is a relative indication but is often considered for stones over about 8mm).

Scenario 1: Ureteric stone

These typically present with acute renal colic symptoms. **Figure 2.7** shows a distal ureteric stone at the VUJ. Strong analgesia is essential and generally NSAIDs are preferred. If a patient presents with a small ureteric stone (<5mm) with no features of sepsis or AKI, and pain is well controlled, then a trial of watchful waiting is reasonable as many stones will pass spontaneously. It is essential that close follow-up of the patient is arranged. Patients may be advised about the chance of their stone passing spontaneously

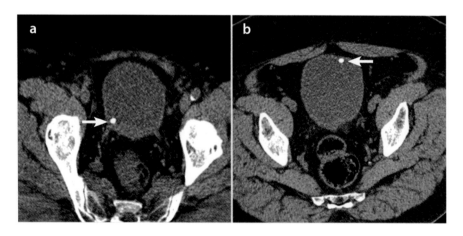

Figure 2.7 Axial non-contrast computed tomography. (**a**) In a supine position with a stone sitting at the right vesicoureteric junction (arrow). This is shown to have actually passed into the bladder on the prone image (**b**) performed at the same time (arrow).

without intervention. Overall, 68% of stones <5mm will pass spontaneously whereas for those >5mm, 47% will pass spontaneously. Overall, 95% of stones <4mm will pass within 40 days[1]. For those patients with stones <10mm (and with no indications for urgent intervention), conservative management with periodic clinical assessment is a suitable initial management option. Generally these patients are reviewed with repeat imaging within 2–3 weeks.

The effectiveness of medical expulsive therapy (e.g. with tamsulosin) has recently been questioned and is no longer offered to patients in many centres[2]. Ureteric stones causing significant obstruction and very high intrarenal pressures may lead to calyceal rupture, urinary extravasation and even urinoma formation (**Figure 2.8**). Insertion of a nephrostomy or ureteric stent may be indicated in this situation. Primary ureteroscopy (that which takes place at or soon after presentation) and laser stone fragmentation or urgent extracorporeal shockwave lithotripsy (ESWL) can also be considered as a treatment for stones that are not expected to pass spontaneously or for those patients in whom conservative management has failed.

Scenario 2: Sepsis with an obstructing stone

This is a urological emergency. The patient should be resuscitated, broad-spectrum intravenous (IV) antibiotics administered and urgent decompression of the infected and obstructed system should be promptly arranged. These patients are acutely unwell and often need management in the critical care setting. Relief of the obstruction can be achieved with retrograde ureteric stent insertion or percutaneous nephrostomy depending upon local arrangements and senior urological input. Often nephrostomy insertion is favoured as it avoids a general anaesthetic, does not increase intrarenal pressures during insertion (which may occur with ureteric stent insertion) and allows monitoring of urine output from the affected kidney. Treating the actual stone is usually deferred until the infection has resolved.

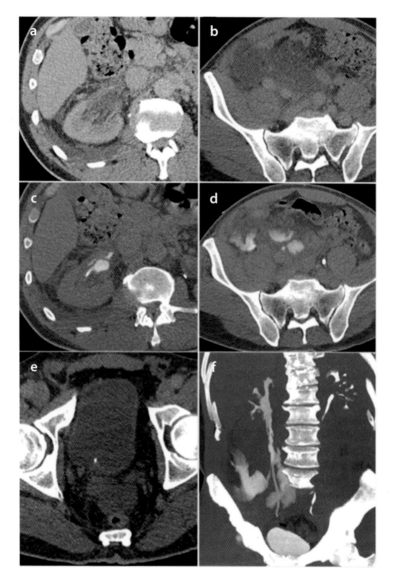

Figure 2.8 Axial computed tomography (CT) images showing: (**a**) inflammatory stranding around the right renal pelvis; (**b**) extensive retroperitoneal fluid tracking down along the right retroperitoneum; (**c**) delayed phase CT showing small amounts of excreted contrast medium outside the renal pelvis; axial and coronal delayed phase (**d**) and (**f**) showing excreted contrast medium in a large retroperitoneal urinoma – all caused by a small right vesicoureteric stone (**e**).

Scenario 3: Staghorn calculi

These are large stones that grow to occupy the renal collecting system (**Figures 2.9, 2.10**). They are most commonly composed of struvite (magnesium ammonium phosphate) and are related to urine infection. They may be detected acutely in a patient with urosepsis or AKI and these must be addressed before management of the stone can be undertaken. Definitive treatment is usually with percutaneous nephrolithotomy (PCNL) surgery. Complications of staghorn stones include renal failure and urosepsis (septicaemia, pyonephrosis or perinephric abscess). Untreated staghorn stones are associated with significant morbidity and mortality.

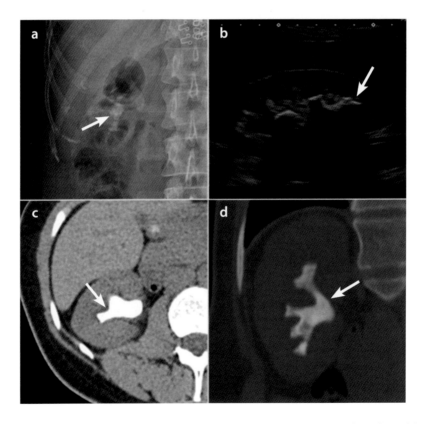

Figure 2.9 A large right staghorn calculus is somewhat obscured by bowel gas on a plain abdominal X-ray (**a**). It is clearly seen on longitudinal ultrasound (**b**) with classical posterior acoustic shadowing and mild dilatation of the upper pole calyx. The staghorn calculus is clearly seen on axial non-contrast computed tomography (**c**) and coronal reconstruction (**d**).

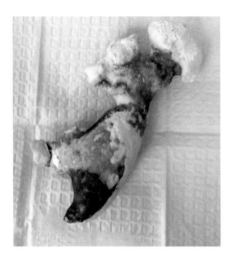

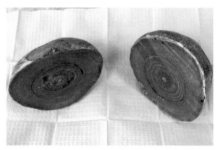

Figure 2.11 A large bladder stone, measuring over 10cm in transverse diameter. This calculus was removed by open cystotomy. It has subsequently been divided to demonstrate its lamina structure.

Figure 2.10 A large staghorn calculus. This calculus was removed in its entirety by an open lithotomy procedure.

Follow-up

The follow-up of patients who present with renal or ureteric stones has several aims:

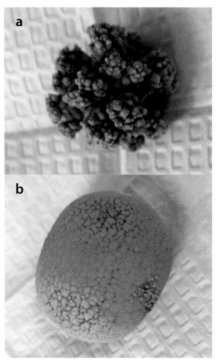

- The first is to ensure that ureteric stones treated conservatively have passed, otherwise, intervention should be arranged (**Figures 2.11, 2.12**).
- If a procedure was undertaken, follow-up is needed to ensure that there has been a good recovery and no complications.
- It is essential that if a ureteric stent has been placed as part of the treatment that plans are in place for its removal.
- Follow-up imaging can ensure effective stone treatment or spontaneous stone passage and can assess for residual stone burden elsewhere in the urinary tract.

Figure 2.12 (**a**) and (**b**) Smaller urinary tract calculi.

Finally, ensure investigations have been undertaken to exclude an underlying predisposition to stone formation. More sophisticated investigations (e.g. full metabolic evaluation with 24-hour urine collections) are reserved for young patients and recurrent stone formers.

All patients should be advised about conservative and dietary measures to prevent future stone formation (particularly maintaining a high fluid intake). Dietary advice is often given to patients to try and reduce their risk of further stone formation. This includes decreasing intake of animal protein (particularly red meat) and avoiding foods that are high in salt and oxalate (as hyperoxaluria predisposes to calcium stone formation), such as spinach, rhubarb and dark chocolate.

Key Points

- Exclude other life-threatening causes of acute-onset pain such as aortic aneurysm.
- Establish early whether the patient has an infected/obstructed kidney, which would require urgent decompression.
- Microscopic haematuria is only about 80% sensitive for ureteric calculi.
- Maintain a ureteric stent register or other method to ensure ureteric stents are not left in patients indefinitely.

KIDNEY INFECTIONS[3]

Pyelonephritis

Pyelonephritis is defined as inflammation of the kidney (renal parenchyma and renal pelvis) – an upper tract UTI.

Acute pyelonephritis is a clinical syndrome associated with characteristic symptoms (of fever, loin pain and commonly nausea and vomiting), whereas chronic pyelonephritis is a radiological diagnosis describing a scarred, shrunken kidney (which may have resulted from recurrent episodes of infection).

Causes

Pyelonephritis is usually caused by the retrograde ascent of urinary pathogens from the lower urinary tract. Therefore, many of the underlying causes and typical causative pathogens are the same as for lower tract UTI (Chapter 3).

As for lower tract UTIs, the pathogenesis results from the interaction of bacterial virulence factors (pyelonephritis is especially associated with the *P. pili* adherence mechanism associated with *E. coli*), susceptibility to infections and host defence mechanisms (e.g. normal antegrade flow of urine/general immune system response). Specific risk factors are outlined in *Box 2.7*.

Presentation

Patients with acute pyelonephritis can vary greatly in the severity of their illness from a mild infection that may be managed in the community with oral antibiotics to an acutely unwell patient with signs of septic shock, who may require high-dependency or intensive-care management.

A key priority in the early management of acutely unwell patients with suspected upper UTI is the detection of, or exclusion of, any obstruction; an infected, obstructed kidney may require urgent decompression with either a nephrostomy or ureteric stent. Again, it is important to consider non-urological causes of acute loin pain, for example, a ruptured AAA that may also present with severe back pain.

Symptoms
- Loin pain.
- Nausea and vomiting.
- Symptoms associated with AKI.
- Fever, confusion (as for lower UTI).
- May have had preceding lower urinary tract symptoms (frequency, urgency, dysuria) suggestive of a lower UTI/ cystitis (which may have already been partially treated) suggesting retrograde ascent of pathogens to the upper tracts.

Box 2.7 Risk factors for pyelonephritis.

- Vesicoureteric reflux.
- Urinary tract obstruction.
- Stones.
- Diabetes/immunosuppression.
- Pregnancy.
- Spinal cord injury (resulting in neuropathic bladder).

Examination
- Routine observation (temperature/ HR/RR/ BP) to diagnose systemic inflammatory response syndrome (SIRS).
- Pyrexia.
- Features of AKI/uraemia.
- Scars suggestive of previous abdominal/pelvic surgery that may predispose to urinary tract obstruction.
- Loin tenderness is a key feature in the examination. Its absence does not exclude an upper tract infection but it may be suggestive of a severe parenchymal infection or pyonephrosis (pus within an obstructed system, requiring urgent decompression).
- Loin mass.
- Abdominal or pelvic mass (including palpable bladder) that may cause upper tract obstruction.
- Presence of catheter (predisposes to infection).

Investigation
- Urine dipstick +/- culture (remember there is a considerable false-negative rate, particularly in those who may have already received antibiotic treatment).
- Bloods (FBC/U&E/CRP/clotting screen: in case an invasive procedure is necessary).
- Blood glucose/HbA1c (if known or suspected diabetes).
- Arterial blood gas if unwell.
- Urgent imaging (ultrasound or CT as first line depending on departmental protocol). **Figure 2.13** demonstrates typical findings on ultrasound and CT scan.

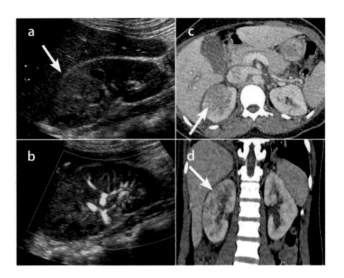

Figure 2.13 Longitudinal ultrasound images of the right kidney (**a**) and (**b**) with power Doppler showing a region of increased echogenicity at the upper pole with reduced vascular flow consistent with pyelonephritis (arrow). Corresponding axial (**c**) and coronal (**d**) portal phase computed tomography images showing patchy reduced cortical perfusion at the right upper pole (arrow) due to pyelonephritis.

Treatment

For those patients who present with a mild, uncomplicated upper tract UTI, the patient may be managed in the community with a 2-week course of antibiotics. The choice of antibiotic should be informed according to local guidelines. The commonest causative pathogens of pyelonephritis are listed in Box 2.8.

If there is any suspicion of a complicated upper tract infection (see below), obstruction, AKI or where patients deteriorate whilst on oral antibiotics, then hospital admission should be arranged for IV antibiotic treatment and other supportive treatments (i.e. decompression of a blocked kidney). For those patients who do not improve after being treated with IV antibiotics whilst in hospital (who may initially have

had reassuring imaging), repeat imaging after 48–72h should be considered to exclude a more severe form of pyelonephritis (e.g. xanthogranulomatous pyelonephritis

Box 2.8 Causative organisms of pyelonephritis (typically Gram-negative).

- E. coli.
- Proteus.
- Klebsiella.
- Pseudomonas.
- Enterobacter.
- Citrobacter.
- Serratia.

and emphysematous pyelonephritis – see later) or the development of a complication such as a renal or peri-renal abscess.

The most important aspect to the management of patients with upper UTIs is to exclude an infected, obstructed kidney. This is a urological emergency. Patients will typically be very unwell, with signs of sepsis and loin pain/tenderness. Urgent senior input, resuscitation, antibiotic treatment and upper tract decompression are needed. The following points refer to the initial management of such patients:

- An initial assessment will identify the acutely unwell patient who should be resuscitated in accordance with national or local resuscitation guidelines and for whom the early involvement of critical care colleagues is important.
- IV fluids.
- IV antibiotics (dictated by local guidelines but ensuring broad-spectrum, Gram-negative and anaerobe cover). Patients are usually treated with IV antibiotics until apyrexial for 24h followed by a 10–14 day course of oral antibiotics. There is a 10–30% relapse rate that usually responds to a further course of antibiotics.
- Optimisation of diabetic control/insulin sliding scale.
- Upper tract decompression (stent or nephrostomy for any infected obstructed kidney).

Follow-up
- A repeat urine culture after treatment is often advocated to ensure successful treatment.
- A single episode of pyelonephritis that settles with a short course of antibiotics does not necessarily require

further investigation. Severe infections, those with a prolonged course or recurrent episodes may warrant further investigation as to an underlying cause.

Specific subtypes of pyelonephritis

Emphysematous pyelonephritis (EPN)
EPN is defined as an acute necrotising parenchymal and peri-renal infection. It is an unusual, severe form of acute pyelonephritis that occurs more often in diabetics. It is associated with gas-forming organisms (especially *E. coli* and *Klebsiella*) (**Figure 2.14**). It presents as a severe form of pyelonephritis that does not respond fully to standard antibiotic treatment.

Resuscitation and IV antibiotic treatment (usually in a critical care setting) is needed with consideration of image-guided drain

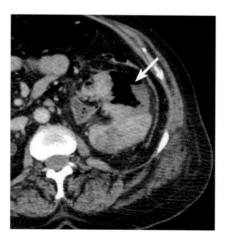

Figure 2.14 Axial portal phase computed tomography image of the left kidney showing emphysematous pyelonephritis with a thick enhancing renal pelvis containing gas along with a cortical gas-containing abscess (arrow).

insertion if there are any collections and an emergency nephrectomy in select cases.

Xanthogranulomatous pyelonephritis (XGP)

XGP is a severe chronic renal infection commonly associated with renal stone disease, resulting in an enlarged and ultimately non-functioning kidney. Risk factors for XGP are lower UTIs, stones, immunosuppression and diabetes mellitus, and it occurs more commonly in females.

Resuscitation and IV antibiotics are the mainstay of therapy with the acute presentation. XGP is difficult to distinguish on imaging from renal cell carcinoma, and once the infection has been treated, patients may go on to have a nephrectomy due to concerns that this may be malignant, when the diagnosis of XGP is then confirmed (**Figure 2.15**).

Renal/peri-renal abscess

Renal abscesses are usually associated with ascending Gram-negative organisms. Patients are usually symptomatic for longer (>5 days) before presenting compared to acute pyelonephritis.

Small renal abscesses (<3cm) may respond to IV antibiotics only; larger ones usually need additional percutaneous drainage. **Figure 2.16** shows the typical appearance of a cortical renal abscess.

Perinephric abscesses refer to pus within Gerota's fascia and the perinephric fat (the outer tissue surrounding the kidney). It usually occurs secondary to pyelonephritis or less often as a result of haematogenous or peri-renal spread (e.g. bowel perforation or Crohn's disease). Treatment is with percutaneous drainage and IV antibiotics.

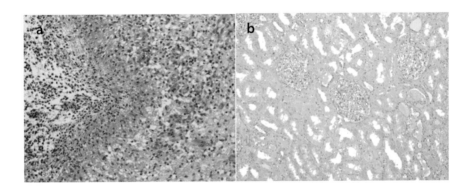

Figure 2.15 (a) and **(b)** Haematoxylin and eosin-stained microscopic images from a kidney with xanthogranulomatous pyelonephritis (XGP). **(a)** Shows an abscess cavity on the left where neutrophils predominate, and adjacent sheets of macrophages (pale staining) on the right. For comparison, **(b)** shows a less inflamed area from the same kidney, where glomeruli (centrally) and renal tubules are preserved. (Images courtesy of Dr Anne Warren.)

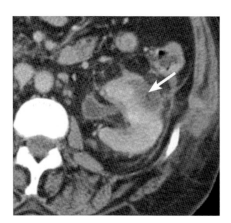

Figure 2.16 Portal phase axial computed tomography image of the left kidney showing enhancement of the renal pelvis in keeping with pyelonephritis that has been complicated by a small cortical abscess (arrow).

Key Points

- Excluding an infected obstructed kidney early is key to the management of patients presenting with suspected pyelonephritis.
- Consider more complicated infections (e.g. renal abscess, EPN, XGP) for those patients that fail to respond to appropriate antibiotic treatment and re-image if necessary.

References

1 Miller OF, Kane CJ. Time to stone passage for observed ureteric calculi. *J Urol* 1999; **162**(3): 688–90.

2 McClinton S, Starr K, Thomas R, *et al*. Use of drug therapy in the management of symptomatic ureteric stones in hospitalized adults (SUSPEND), a multicentre, placebo-controlled, randomized trial of a calcium-channel blocker (nifedipine) and an α-blocker (tamsulosin): study protocol for a randomized controlled trial. *Trials* 2014; **15**: 238–50.

Chapter 3

Lower Urinary Tract Emergencies

David Thurtle and Suzanne Biers[1, 3, 4, 5] / Alexandra Colquhoun[2]

URINARY RETENTION[1]

Acute urinary retention (AUR) is the painful inability to pass urine (void). It is followed by relief of pain on catheterisation with good urine volume output.

Chronic urinary retention (CUR) is less well defined, but importantly is not painful and the patient continues to void (this may or may not be 'normal' voiding). Older definitions described a palpable/percussable bladder after voiding. The National Institute for Health and Care Excellence (NICE) defines CUR as a post-void residual volume of >1000ml (other definitions suggest smaller volumes and in fact any patient that does not empty their bladder completely might be considered to be retaining urine).

Acute or chronic urinary retention is a new inability to pass urine on a background of CUR.

Anuria is defined as the passage of less than 50ml urine in 1 day. Provided obstruction has been excluded, it is a sign of acute kidney injury (AKI), and requires medical referral and input (see Chapter 2).

Acute urinary retention

AUR is much more common in men than women. Between 4% and 7% of men will experience AUR at some point in their life. Although prostatic pathology is by far the most common, AUR has numerous causes. Broadly, AUR is due to either obstruction to the urine leaving the bladder or reduced/ineffective bladder contractility. The most common causes of bladder outlet obstruction (BOO) in men are shown in *Box 3.1*, and in women in *Box 3.2*. Causes of reduced bladder contractility can be similar in both

Box 3.1 Male causes of BOO.

- Benign prostatic enlargement (BPE).
- Malignant enlargement of the prostate.
- Urethral stricture.
- Clot retention.
- Urethral stone.
- Urinary tract infection (UTI)/prostatitis.
- Constipation.
- Neurological.

Box 3.2 Female causes of BOO.

- Pelvic organ prolapse.
- Urethral stricture.
- Clot retention.
- Urethral diverticulum.
- After stress incontinence surgery.
- UTI.
- Fowler's syndrome (impaired sphincter relaxation).
- Constipation.
- Pelvic mass/tumour.
- Neurological.

Box 3.3 Causes of reduced bladder contractility.

- Drugs (*see Box 3.4*).
- Episode of overdistension of bladder.
- Sacral or cauda equina nerve compression or injury.
- Supra-sacral spinal cord injury.
- Pelvic surgery/pelvic fracture (due to autonomic nerve damage).
- Infection.
- Multiple sclerosis.
- Diabetes mellitus (sensory and motor dysfunction).
- Post-operative (immobility/anaesthetic agents/analgesics/epidural/pelvic or abdominal surgery).

sexes (*Boxes 3.3* and *3.4*). AUR can also be classified as 'spontaneous' or 'precipitated'. Spontaneous retention is something of a misnomer as there remains a cause, often benign prostatic enlargement, but the term is used when no obvious precipitating cause is found.

Presentation

Classically, patients report suprapubic pain and an inability to pass urine, which may be associated with a recent onset or deterioration of urinary symptoms. A full urological history will help to define the cause, once the retention has been drained.

History
- Duration of onset (usually hours).
- Preceding lower urinary tract symptoms (LUTS): patients usually describe worsening symptoms over days.

- Any fever or dysuria (indicates infective cause).
- Precipitating factors (constipation, general anaesthesia, recent surgery, e.g. haemorrhoidectomy, inguinal hernia, orthopaedic surgery).
- Associated flank pain or a history of nocturnal incontinence (may suggest high pressure chronic retention causing hydronephrosis).
- Ask about back pain and neurological symptoms.
- Any visible haematuria.
- Drug history: recent new medications (e.g. drugs with anticholinergic effects can cause urinary retention directly or by causing constipation), medication acting on the prostate to relieve bladder outflow obstruction,

Box 3.4 Pharmacological agents increasing the risk of urinary retention.

- Antimuscarinics:
  - › Oxybutynin.
  - › Solifenacin.
  - › Atropine.
  - › Hyoscine butylbromide.
- Antihistamines:
  - › Chlorpheniramine.
  - › Diphenhydramine.
- Sympathomimetics:
  - › Oral decongestants.
- Antipsychotics.
- Antiparkinsonian agents.
- Muscle relaxants.
- Opioid analgesics.

anticoagulant medication (must be considered if suprapubic catheter insertion is needed).
- Previous medical history: history of pelvic or prostate cancer, post-menopausal bleeding (may indicate pelvic pathology in females), any recent urinary tract surgery.

Examination
- AUR patients are in obvious discomfort.
- Tender, palpable, percussable bladder suprapubically.
- Digital rectal examination (after emptying the bladder) to assess the prostate size and contour for cancer, and assess for constipation or rectal masses.
- Assess neurology, anal tone and peri-anal sensation if indicated.
- Bimanual vaginal exam to assess for pelvic masses.

Investigation
- A handheld bladder ultrasound scan (USS) may be useful to check the bladder volume if there is any uncertainty about the diagnosis.
- Dipstick urinalysis +/- culture (following sterile catheter insertion, or suprapubic aspiration).
- Check urea and electrolytes (U&E), full blood count (FBC), C-reactive protein (CRP) +/- blood cultures. Venous blood gas for urgent potassium level.
- USS of the renal tract should be considered where upper tract dysfunction is suspected (e.g. elevated creatinine).
- Magnetic resonance imaging (MRI) of the spine should be performed urgently if there are any concerns of acute spinal injury.
- Prostate-specific antigen (PSA) blood test is deferred as it can be abnormally raised with AUR or by catheterisation.

Management
In all cases of AUR, the first priority is urgent relief of retention. Attempt urethral catheterisation first (see page 151 'catheter skills' for tips). If this is unsuccessful, request advice or assessment from a urologist who will have the expertise and access to alternative catheter types (e.g. curved tip catheters such as Coudé or Tiemann), flexible cystoscopy and guidewire insertion of a catheter +/- urethral dilatation. Suprapubic catheter insertion using ultrasound guidance is an alternative if there are no patient contraindications (see page 153). Use a urometer drainage bag that can accurately record urine output.

Record in the medical case notes the volume immediately drained from the bladder, and ask for urine output to then be recorded hourly initially to exclude diuresis. Further management depends on the underlying cause of retention as outlined below.

Benign prostatic enlargement

- Immediate: start an alpha-blocker (tamsulosin 400μg daily). A trial without catheter (TWOC) can be considered after 2–3 days, though it is not always successful (*Box 3.5*).
- Delayed: additional drugs (e.g. 5-alpha-reductase inhibitors, *Box 3.6*) can be added if there is a persistent failure to void or persistent obstructive voiding symptoms after the catheter is removed. Finasteride, a 5-alpha-reductase inhibitor (5-ARI), reduces the volume of the prostate by about 25% but it takes many months before a patient derives its maximal clinical effect. Most men who fail to void after catheter removal will be considered for bladder outflow surgery such as a transurethral resection of the prostate (TURP) (**Figure 3.1**) or holmium laser enucleation of the prostate (HoLEP) (**Figure 3.2**). Clean intermittent self-catheterisation (CISC) or a long-term indwelling catheter are alternatives. In exceptional circumstances, e.g. medically unfit patients, a further attempt at catheter removal may be attempted after several months of treatment with a 5-ARI.

Box 3.5 Rates of recurrence of retention in men.

Precipitated retention

- Once the precipitant is treated/removed, it is uncommon to get a second episode unless underlying risk factors are present.
- Delaying TWOC to 7 days can increase the chance of success.

'Spontaneous' retention

- 50% recurrence within 1 week.
- 70% within 1 year (without treatment).

Retention related to BPE

- 60% of men treated with 1–3 days of an alpha-blocker were able to void spontaneously post-TWOC, compared to 38% on placebo[1].
- Recurrent acute retention incidence is 31% lower in those treated with an alpha-blocker[1].

Box 3.6 Medication for BPH.

- Alpha-blockers (tamsulosin/alfuzosin):
  › Block alpha-1 adrenergic receptors in smooth muscles, including in the prostate.
  › Patients should be warned of retrograde ejaculation or 'dry orgasm'.
  › Can cause hypotension and dizziness, although tamsulosin is the most selective to prostatic α-1a adrenergic receptors.
  › Onset of action within days.
- 5-alpha-reductase inhibitors (finasteride/dutasteride):
  › Block the enzyme that converts testosterone to more potent androgens (dihydrotestosterone/DHT), which are promoters of prostatic growth.
  › Takes up to 6 months for maximal therapeutic benefit.
  › May negatively affect sexual function (loss of libido and impotence).
  › Will half PSA levels after 6 months.

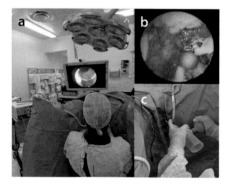

Figure 3.1 Surgical option for treating bladder outlet obstruction in men. Intra-operative images of transurethral resection of the prostate (TURP). Surgeon operating with a monopolar TURP resecting loop (a), roller-ball diathermy (b), evacuation of prostatic chips with an Ellik evacuator (c).

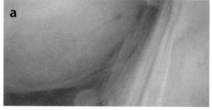

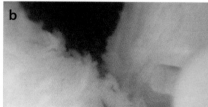

Figure 3.2 Surgical option for treating bladder outlet obstruction in men. Intra-operative pictures of holmium laser enucleation of the prostate (HoLEP). The plane of the prostatic capsule is being developed (a). Laser incision through the hyperplastic prostate with the bladder visible above (b). Note how little haemorrhage is evident. (Images courtesy of Mr Tev Aho.)

Clot retention

- Immediate: 3-way catheter (>20 Fr) insertion, bladder washout and saline irrigation. Treat any related cause (i.e. check for and treat abnormal clotting; treat any infection) (see page 52 for haematuria).
- Delayed: haematuria needs full investigation with flexible cystoscopy under local anaesthesia when the urine is clear, imaging of the urinary tract (USS urinary tract or computed tomography [CT] urogram) and often urine cytology also.

Urethral stricture

- Immediate: often it is not evident the patient has a stricture until it is difficult to pass a urethral catheter. In the emergency setting, urologists will often still attempt gentle catheterisation with a smaller calibre and stiffer material device (such as a silicone 12 Fr catheter), although any force should be avoided as this can cause false passages in the urethra. If this fails, alternative techniques include urethral dilatation and insertion of a urethral catheter or insertion of a suprapubic catheter.
- Delayed: formal urethral dilatation under anaesthesia, optical urethrotomy (opening up of urethral stricture using a fine blade) or urethroplasty (excision of stricture and reconstruction of the urethra, sometimes using the buccal mucosa of the cheek as graft tissue).

UTI

Management is discussed on page 61. If the patient has had recent instrumentation/surgery, give prophylactic antibiotics to cover catheter insertion.

Constipation

Treat with either suppositories or enemas and oral laxatives. Remember, constipation may be a sign of a neurological pathology. Attempt TWOC after the bowels have been fully evacuated.

Neurological

- Remove or treat the offending cause.
- Do not miss neurological injuries: consider cauda equina syndrome (see page 121 for neurological topics).

Chronic urinary retention

Patients with CUR are less likely to present to the emergency department. However, a grossly enlarged bladder is not an uncommon finding in a primary care doctor's surgery or in the urology outpatient department. The patient may be referred for acute or elective hospital review due to a palpable bladder or develop acute on chronic urinary retention and present as an emergency.

CUR can be subdivided into low-pressure or high-pressure conditions. Low-pressure CUR is caused predominantly by primary detrusor (bladder muscle) failure and does not tend to cause obstructive uropathy. In high-pressure CUR (HPCUR) the detrusor attempts to compensate for the increased outflow resistance with hypertrophy. A thickened, fibrous, trabeculated bladder wall develops over time, resulting in a raised intravesical pressure leading to hydronephrosis (**Figure 3.3**) and bladder diverticula. When detrusor pressure can no longer overcome the obstruction to voiding or there is an acute precipitating event, patients may present with acute on chronic retention.

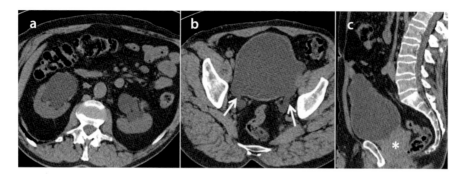

Figure 3.3 A male patient presenting with urinary retention and acute kidney injury. Axial non-contrast computed tomography (CT) images (**a**) of the kidneys showing bilateral hydronephrosis, and (**b**) of a full bladder with dilated distal ureters (white arrows) with widely patent vesicoureteric junctions; (**c**) sagittal CT image showing a large-volume bladder extending nearly up to the umbilicus due to a large prostate (asterisk).

Symptoms

- Nocturnal enuresis (incontinence at night whilst asleep), as the bladder pressure exceeds the relaxed urethral pressure overnight.
- LUTS, especially nocturia and sensation of incomplete bladder emptying.
- Sensation of abdominal bloating/fullness.
- Patients with HPCUR may report a history of hypertension, renal impairment or congestive cardiac failure.
- Recurrent UTIs as a result of urinary stasis.
- Bilateral flank pain may suggest HPCUR.

Investigation

As per AUR – renal function, residual volume measurement and urgent upper tract imaging are particularly important in HPCUR. Note, it is not uncommon for hydronephrosis to persist for some time after decompression of the bladder. Improving renal function should provide reassurance, and an USS may be repeated after several days to assess resolution.

Management

- Immediate:
  › Catheterisation.
  › Monitor urine output closely. Greater than 200ml urine output per hour for >2–4 hours suggests post-obstructive diuresis (see further management below).
  › Post-decompression haematuria is not uncommon. This is usually a self-limiting condition, only requiring treatment if severe and causing clot retention. A silicone catheter or wide-bore urethral catheter (i.e. 16 Fr or 18 Fr) can be used pre-emptively as these are less likely to become blocked and can be more easily flushed in the event of post-decompression bleeding.

- Delayed:
  › HPCUR patients should not have a TWOC and will require bladder outlet surgery if they are fit enough. A long-term catheter will be required otherwise.
  › 'Low-pressure' CUR patients often require urodynamic studies to guide treatment. Bladder outlet surgery is generally not effective for patients with detrusor failure as the bladder cannot generate a sufficient contraction to expel urine. Instead these patients require bladder drainage via an intermittent or indwelling catheter.

Post-obstructive diuresis

Post-obstructive diuresis is thought to result from the physiological excretion of the chronically retained urea, sodium and water. Furthermore, the corticomedullary gradient is lost in the obstructed kidney and the kidney is unable to immediately adjust when the obstruction is relieved. This diuresis may also be indicative of a persistent tubular dysfunction with an inadequate response to antidiuretic hormone (ADH).

Management
- Requires admission and observation.
- Hourly urine output.
- Daily U&E initially (watch for hyponatraemia).
- Daily weights.
- Lying/standing blood pressure (BP) (to assess for significant postural drop).
- Supplement with intravenous (IV) fluids (usually saline) if there is inadequate oral intake. Overall, aim to replace fluids at around 50% of the previous hour's urine output.

- U&E should be repeated over the following weeks and months to ensure recovery in renal function.

Retention with catheterisable stomas

Patients with catheterisable stomas, such as Mitrofanoffs (appendix used as a catheterisable vesicocutaneous channel as an alternative route to perform clean intermittent self-catheterisation [CISC]) may present with retention due to failure to insert a catheter into the channel to drain the bladder. Urology input is required. It is reasonable for a urologist to attempt gentle catheterisation, with plenty of anaesthetic lubricant jelly and a small-calibre catheter (10–12 Fr guided by the patient's usual catheter size). If this fails, enlist help from interventional radiology, who can try passing a hydrophilic guide-wire under fluoroscopic guidance, perform gentle dilation of the channel, and follow with Seldinger insertion of an open tip catheter over the wire (**Figure 3.4**). If the urethra is patent and accessible, a temporary urethral catheter can be placed to relieve acute retention.

Important

It is not safe to remove the catheter of a patient with HPCUR (associated with renal impairment). These patients will require bladder outflow surgery or long-term catheterisation to avoid kidney damage.

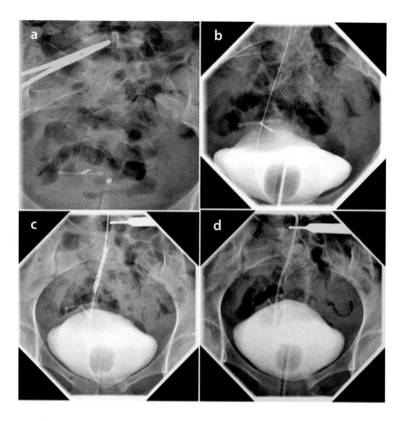

Figure 3.4 A patient with a Mitrofanoff channel from the umbilicus to the bladder, who presented with difficulty performing self-catheterisation down the channel. Fluoroscopic images: (**a**) metal forceps pointing to the umbilical opening; (**b**) showing bladder filling along with a wire inserted through the Mitrofanoff; (**c**) with contrast medium injected along a tight Mitrofanoff channel; (**d**) with a pigtail catheter inserted through the Mitrofanoff into the bladder from emergency treatment of retention to assist bladder drainage.

Key Points

- AUR is painful – drain the bladder urgently.
- Always check biochemistry, record bladder volume and monitor early urine output.
- Assess for reversible causes of retention and treat them.
- Be vigilant for HPCUR and acute neurological conditions.

HAEMATURIA[2]

Haematuria is the presence of blood in the urine.

Haematuria is either appreciable to the naked eye, visible haematuria, or detectable on urine dipstick testing, non-visible haematuria (*Table 3.1*).

Table 3.1 Classification of haematuria.

Visible	Non-visible
Appreciable to the naked eye	Present on urine dipstick
Synonyms: • Frank • Gross • Macroscopic	Synonyms: • Dipstick • Invisible • Microscopic

Visible haematuria is an alarming symptom and often prompts emergency or urgent presentation to either primary or secondary care. Management and further investigation of haematuria is important as a high proportion of patients will have sinister or serious pathology accounting for the presence of blood in the urine.

Non-visible haematuria is defined as a positive urine dipstick measuring at least 1+ on the dipstick scale. 'Trace' dipstick haematuria is not considered significant and does not warrant further investigation. Urine microscopy is less sensitive than urine dipstick testing due to a high false-negative rate and is not recommended to determine the presence of non-visible haematuria.

Causes

Haematuria has many causes some of which are easily treatable (e.g. UTI) and some of which require more complex intervention (e.g. muscle-invasive bladder cancer). A comprehensive list of the causes of haematuria is shown in *Table 3.2*. The more common causes can be grouped as follows:

- Urological malignancy, including bladder cancer (**Figure 3.5**), renal cancer (**Figure 3.6**) and prostate cancer.

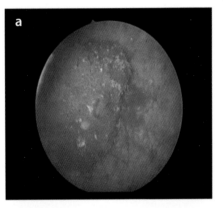

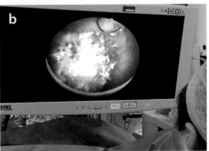

Figure 3.5 Cystoscopic view of a solitary bladder cancer (**a**) and transurethral resection of the bladder tumour with a resectoscope using a wire loop (**b**).

Table 3.2 Causes of haematuria.

Neoplastic	Prostate Kidney Bladder Ureteric Penile
Infective	UTI Prostatitis Urethritis Epididymo-orchitis Tuberculosis Schistosomiasis
Mechanical	Calculi (renal, ureteric, bladder) Strictures (PUJO, ureteric, urethral) Trauma Benign prostatic enlargement
Nephrological	Glomerular bleeding: • IgA nephropathy • Alport's nephritis • Systemic lupus erythematosus • Goodpasture's syndrome • Glomerulonephritis: streptococcal, mesangioproliferative, mesangiocapillary and membranous types Medullary sponge kidney Polycystic kidney disease Arteriovenous fistula/malformation Renal artery embolism/thrombosis Papillary necrosis
Miscellaneous	Radiation cystitis Coagulopathy: • Thrombocytopaenia • Haemophilia • DIC • Drug-induced coagulopathy Exercise/march haematuria Paroxysmal nocturnal haematuria
Non-haematuria*	Drugs: • Rifampicin • Sulfasalazine • Metronidazole • Nitrofurantoin Menstruation Anthrocyanin ingestion (beetroot/blackberries)

*Non-haematuria or false positives for haematuria due to altered urinary colour or false-positive dipstick urinalysis.
DIC: disseminated intravascular coagulopathy; PUJO: pelviureteric junction obstruction; UTI: urinary tract infection.

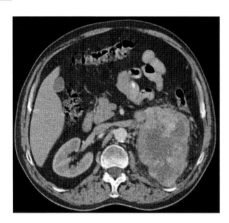

Figure 3.6 An axial image of a computed tomography scan with contrast demonstrating a left renal cell carcinoma.

- UTI, including common uropathogens such as *Escherichia coli*, or rarer micro-organisms including those causing schistosomiasis or tuberculosis.
- Calculus disease, either renal/ureteric calculi or bladder stones (**Figure 3.7**).
- Urethral stricture disease.

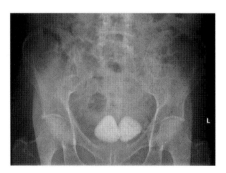

Figure 3.7 A plain pelvic X-ray demonstrating two large stones in the bladder.

Managing patients in the emergency setting

Perform an initial rapid assessment and resuscitate the patient if there is evidence of haemodynamic instability. When the patient is stable, a full assessment can proceed. The majority of patients presenting in the emergency setting will have visible haematuria. History taking should cover the following salient points: duration and severity of haematuria, presence of clots, associated pain (loin or suprapubic), systemic upset (fever), history of trauma and any associated LUTS. Medication history should determine anticoagulant usage and social history should ascertain smoking status and (former) occupation. General examination should determine haemodynamic stability and assess for stigmata of anaemia. Focused abdominal examination should determine the presence of a full bladder (clot retention), loin masses or tenderness, and examination of both the external genitalia and prostate are mandatory. A summary of the initial assessment is outlined in *Table 3.3*.

Further management is dependent on the preceding history. Baseline investigations routinely include urine culture (if the haematuria is not too excessive), blood testing including FBC, renal and liver function, bone profile and a group and save/cross-match if potential transfusion is anticipated.

Table 3.3 Emergency assessment of haematuria.

History	
• Duration of bleeding	• Associated LUTS
• Severity:	• Use of anticoagulants:
› Mild	› Aspirin
› Moderate	› Clopidogrel
› Heavy	› Warfarin
• Presence of clots	› Heparin
• Associated pain:	› Novel oral anticoagulants (e.g. dabigatran/rivaroxaban)
› Loin	• Smoking status
› Suprapubic	• Occupation

Examination	
• Haemodynamic stability	• Digital rectal examination:
• Presence of anaemia	› Prostate cancer
• Palpable bladder	› BPE
• Palpable loin mass	• Female pelvic exam if indicated (i.e. post-menopausal bleeding; concern that reported visible blood may originate from vagina)
• Examine external genitalia:	
› Phimosis	
› Epididymo-orchitis	

Initial investigations
• MSU
• Bloods:
› FBC
› U&E
› LFT
› Clotting screen
› Group and save/cross-match

BPE: Benign prostatic enlargement; FBC: full blood count; LFT: liver function tests; LUTS: lower urinary tract symptoms; MSU: mid-stream urine; U&E: urea and electrolytes.

Bladder washout for clot retention

Patients with clot retention should be catheterised with a 3-way catheter and irrigation established prior to arranging admission to hospital. A 3-way catheter is inserted using the same aseptic no touch technique employed for all catheterisation procedures (see Chapter 7). In general, 3-way catheters have a larger diameter (usually >20 Ch) to permit passage of clots, and it is often helpful to use two tubes of instillation lubricant to aid insertion. Irrigation (with normal saline) is connected to the in-flow channel of the 3-way catheter using a urology irrigation giving set.

If the bladder contains a large volume of clot, a manual washout may be required in order to establish flow of the irrigant. This is achieved using normal saline and a bladder syringe; the equipment required is shown in **Figure 3.8**. Approximately 50ml of sterile normal saline is gently injected into the bladder through the catheter out-flow channel. A further 50ml is gently injected, then 50ml is very gently syringed back out of the bladder along with any small clots (if 50ml is simply inserted and withdrawn, the bladder mucosa can be drawn in, making washout more difficult). The procedure is repeated several times until no further clot can be extracted from the bladder. The procedure is sometimes easier to achieve with the catheter balloon deflated and an assistant holding the catheter in position to prevent dislodgement. The key to an effective bladder washout is not to exert sudden changes in pressure as this can generate a split in the bladder wall and is also extremely painful for a patient in clot retention. If irrigation cannot be established after manual bladder washout, the patient may require bladder washout under general anaesthesia. This is achieved

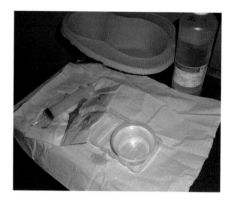

Figure 3.8 The equipment required for a manual bladder washout, in a patient who already has a wide-calibre catheter *in situ*. A sterile bowl or jug is used to draw up the saline, with the resulting bladder aspirate or clots discarded into a non-sterile container.

using the same technique as a manual bladder washout but is performed after inserting the outer sheath of an irrigating cystoscope (24–28 Ch) into the urethra, which permits extraction of larger clots. Such procedures carry a significant risk of bladder perforation and should only be carried out by experienced urologists.

Further investigation and management of acute presentation of haematuria

Other indications for acute admission to hospital include a history of trauma, concomitant usage of anticoagulants and haematuria associated with loin pain (*Table 3.4*). Patients who have sustained trauma and have visible haematuria should have urgent CT-based imaging in the emergency department. Any active source of bleeding (usually from the kidney) should be treated by selective embolisation (see Chapter 8). Patients who are not actively bleeding

Table 3.4 Indications for hospital admission with visible haematuria.

Indication	Rationale
Clot retention	To establish catheter drainage +/- irrigation
Associated trauma	To permit observation for haemodynamic instability
Use of anticoagulation	To reverse any coagulopathy if feasible and appropriate
Associated loin pain	To exclude or treat an infected obstructed kidney; to treat clot colic

should be admitted for bed rest and close observation of haemodynamic parameters. Patients who are anticoagulated should have a clotting screen performed and, if feasible and appropriate (i.e. those whose anticoagulation is not imperative), the anticoagulation should be reversed. The current range of anticoagulation medication available is broad and not all anticoagulants have a reversal agent. Early discussion with colleagues in haematology is recommended if the patient is using an unfamiliar anticoagulant. Patients who have visible haematuria and associated loin pain should be assessed for potential infected obstructed kidneys or a possible bleeding renal lesion causing clot colic. Clot colic is acutely painful and like renal colic is managed with adequate analgesia and prompt investigation of the underlying cause.

During an inpatient stay, imaging of the upper tracts should be arranged (either a triple-phase CT if renal function permits, or renal tract ultrasound and plain X-ray of the kidneys, ureters, bladder [KUB] if renal function is impaired) if possible. If hospital admission is not warranted or early discharge feasible, urgent outpatient-based imaging should be arranged. Flexible cystoscopy will also be required, but is often best deferred to an urgent outpatient basis when the haematuria has resolved so that optimum views of the bladder can be achieved.

Managing patients in primary care

Haematuria, both visible and non-visible, is a common presenting symptom in primary care and not all patients require investigation. Epidemiological studies in the primary care setting indicate 1–2% of patients with haematuria are ultimately found to have sinister urological pathology, e.g. bladder cancer[2]. Conversely, 15% of patients attending secondary care haematuria clinics are found to harbour urological cancer of some form[3], indicating primary care doctors are adept at risk stratification. In addition to referral to urology, referral to nephrology should also be considered for patients with non-visible haematuria (especially if there is associated protein on urine dipstick, renal impairment and also when a urological cause has been excluded).

Patients with haematuria in whom urological cancer is suspected require referral on a 2-week wait basis. The current 2-week wait referral criteria for haematuria are defined in the 2015 UK NICE guidance on suspected cancer[4] and include:

- Unexplained visible haematuria without UTI in a patient over 45 years of age.
- Visible haematuria that persists or recurs after successful treatment of UTI, in a patient over 45 years of age.
- Unexplained non-visible haematuria and either dysuria or a raised white cell count on a blood test, in a patient over 60 years of age.

Patients with visible or non-visible haematuria not fulfilling these categories where a urological cause is suspected should be referred to the urology outpatient clinic on an urgent basis. If a nephrological cause is suspected, the joint British Association of Urological Surgeons and Renal Association guidelines[5] recommend referral to nephrology for anyone not fulfilling criteria for urological assessment especially if there is:

- Declining estimated glomerular filtration rate.
- Significant proteinuria (albumin creatinine ratio ≥30mg/mmol).
- Associated hypertension under the age of 40.
- Associated upper respiratory tract infection.

Investigations commonly undertaken within the haematuria clinic include:

- Urine dipstick and culture.
- Urine cytology.
- Local anaesthetic flexible cystoscopy.
- Upper tract imaging: for visible haematuria, a triple-phase CT; for non-visible haematuria, ultrasound +/- plain KUB X-ray.

Key Points

- Ensure the patient is stable and resuscitate if there is any evidence of haemodynamic compromise.
- Treat clot retention with a large-calibre 3-way catheter and perform a gentle bladder washout to evacuate clot prior to starting irrigation.
- Remember to check if the patient is on anticoagulation, and stop or reverse this (if clinically indicated) in the acute setting under haematology guidance.
- Investigate the underlying cause of the haematuria and refer on for appropriate treatment.

URINARY TRACT INFECTION AND CYSTITIS[3]

A urinary tract infection (UTI) is the presence of, and inflammatory response to, micro-organisms in the urine and is classically defined as bacterial infection of the urine with $>10^5$ colony-forming units (CFU)/ml of mid-stream urine (MSU). Patients can have UTI/bacteriuria with lower values of CFUs, but laboratories may not report these. On suprapubic aspirate, any bacterial growth is significant.

UTIs can be classified by their anatomical location (*Box 3.7*). Upper tract UTIs are discussed in Chapter 2. UTIs can also be classified as 'uncomplicated' or 'complicated'. UTIs are complicated when an underlying risk factor, anatomical, or functional abnormality is also present.

UTIs affect 3% of women annually, 15% of whom have recurrent UTIs. Approximately 50% of females will have a UTI at some point in their life. This represents a significant disease burden and inevitably means presentations of UTI to primary and secondary care are common. Importantly, UTIs are also the most common hospital-acquired infection.

Acute bacterial cystitis

Acute inflammation of the bladder in response to bacteria in the urine.

Causes

Both patient-related and organism-related factors influence the causation of UTI. Antegrade urinary flow, effective sphincters, a well-functioning immune system and other host factors such as protective vaginal commensal bacteria ordinarily help to prevent UTIs. Therefore, damage to these mechanisms increases

Box 3.7 Classification of UTIs.

- Uncomplicated lower tract UTI: cystitis (acute, sporadic or recurrent).
- Uncomplicated upper tract UTI: pyelonephritis (acute, sporadic, no risk factor identified).
- Complicated UTI with or without pyelonephritis (underlying urological, nephrological or other risk factors).
- Urethritis.
- Male accessory gland infection (MAGI): prostatitis, epididymitis, orchitis.

the likelihood of infection, for example with obstruction, catheterisation, immuno-compromise and vaginal atrophy, respectively. *Box 3.8* lists other patient-related factors increasing the likelihood and risk of UTIs. It would be reasonable to refer to a UTI in the context of any of these factors as a 'complicated' infection.

'Obstruction' is an umbrella term that should be linked with an anatomical site such as BOO, where inadequate emptying and urinary stasis can pre-dispose to UTI. BPE is the predominant cause of BOO and for this reason, the proportion of UTIs in male patients increases significantly with age.

Most UTIs are caused by bacteria from the gastrointestinal tract, with approximately 80% due to *E. coli*. With its pili and fimbriae, *E. coli* is able to attach itself to the urothelium of the bladder and upper urinary tract. This virulence mechanism enables the bacteria to ascend causing

Box 3.8 Patient-related factors in risk of UTI.

- Catheter.
- Foreign body (e.g. artificial urinary sphincter, penile prosthesis).
- Instrumentation/surgery.
- Stones.
- Obstruction.
- Reflux.
- Diabetes.
- Immunocompromise.
- Pregnancy.
- Post-menopausal atrophic vaginitis.

Box 3.9 Common causative organisms of acute bacterial cystitis.

Gram −ve
- *E. coli.*
- *Klebsiella sp.*
- *Enterobacter sp.*
- *Proteus sp.*
- *Pseudomonas sp.*

Gram +ve
- *Staphylococcus sp.*
- *Enterococcus sp.*

upper tract UTIs and resist being flushed away. Other causative organisms are listed, in approximate order of prevalence, in *Box 3.9*. Like many infections, the causative organisms in hospitalised patients can be different from those in the community, with Gram-positive bacteria more commonly found in the urine of hospitalised patients. Although the listed bacteria are the most common pathogens, always consider patient-related factors or events that may pre-dispose to alternative pathogens, such as anaerobes following bowel surgery, *Staphylococcus* if a communication is present with the skin or wound, and even atypical organisms such as *Mycobacterium* if the patient has a history of tuberculosis. *Proteus* species are often found in patients with urinary tract stones or foreign material in the urinary tract.

Presentation

The spectrum of presentations for lower tract UTIs is varied, ranging from troublesome new urinary frequency presenting to a primary care doctor, to severe septic shock presenting to the emergency department. Patient factors, mechanical factors and organism factors (multi-resistant strains, virulence) will each influence the risk of developing sepsis (Chapter 1, page 12). Try to establish a trigger or underlying cause (i.e. recent urological intervention, presence of a catheter, stone history, previous recurrent UTIs). Regardless, the focus should be on early recognition and appropriate goal-directed management.

Symptoms

- LUTS: urinary frequency, urgency, dysuria, with offensive smelling urine and pain.
- Fever, lethargy, confusion (especially in the elderly).
- Altered urine colour or clarity +/- haematuria, debris or blocked catheter.

- Loin pain, fever and nausea (with a positive urine dipstick) are typical of pyelonephritis.

Examination
- Observations: pyrexia is common; rigors suggest sepsis.
- Suprapubic tenderness.
- Examine the genitalia for tenderness or swelling or the epididymis or testis. Is a catheter *in situ*?
- Digital rectal examination (DRE): prostate volume, is the prostate tender, warm or boggy (this may represent an abscess)?
- Examine the flanks for tenderness or a palpable mass.
- Look in the catheter bag if present. Is it draining? Is the urine cloudy, blood stained or particularly malodorous?

Investigation
- Dipstick urinalysis (*Table 3.5*).
- Urine culture (to definitively diagnose and later direct antibiotic therapy).
- Post-void residual (PVR) bladder scan (**Figure 3.9**). If this demonstrates a significant urinary volume in the presence of a UTI, this may require catheter drainage.
- FBC and CRP to assess for inflammatory response; U&E to rule out associated AKI; glucose; arterial blood gas (ABG) if systemically unwell.
- USS KUB is the best first-line investigation if pyelonephritis is suspected. It may confirm the diagnosis and exclude hydronephrosis.
- CT KUB is the investigation of choice if there is any suspicion of stones.

Management
- Immediate/short-term:
  › Resuscitate: ABCDE approach (see page 185) and 'Surviving Sepsis Bundle' (page 14).
  › Treat any nidus of infection or reversible cause.
  › Drain/catheterise the bladder if there is a high PVR.

Table **3.5** Dipstick urinalysis in UTI.

	Sensitivity for UTI
Nitrite +	54–90%
Leucocyte +	53–86%
Nitrite + Leuc +	75–96%
No abnormality in up to 20%	

Beware of false negatives, especially in very concentrated/dark urine.

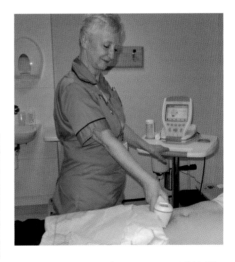

Figure 3.9 Nurse performing a post-void bladder scan with a handheld device.

> › Remove/bypass any foreign object or stone (**Figures 3.10, 3.11**).
> › IV empirical antibiotics as per local guidelines until a urine culture result is available.
> › IV fluids and supportive management.
> › Optimise diabetic control.
> › Switch to oral antibiotics once well/ or start with oral antibiotics if stable (*Box 3.10*).

- Longer-term/follow-up:
  - › Clinical review and dipstick urinalysis are sufficient follow-up in females with uncomplicated UTIs.
  - › If UTIs 'recur' within 2 weeks of treatment with the correct antibiotic, this suggests bacterial persistence; often this is caused by an underlying anatomical or functional abnormality. Repeat the urine culture and arrange urinary tract evaluation.

Box 3.10 Duration of antibiotics.

- Acute uncomplicated cystitis: 3–5 days.
- (Febrile) complicated UTI with urological complicating factors: 7–14 days.
- Pyelonephritis: 10–14 days; switch from IV to oral therapy once sensitivities are known.
- Consider the combination of two antibiotics in severe infections.
- Where interventions are required for infection control, continue antibiotics for 3–5 days after intervention.

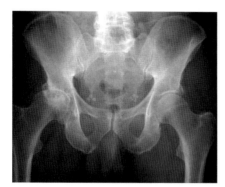

Figure 3.10 Plain film of the pelvis with numerous bladder stones, a cause of bacterial persistence.

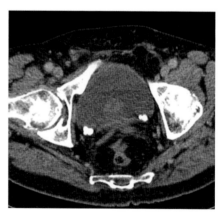

Figure 3.11 Axial computed tomography (CT) image of the bladder showing multiple bladder stones displaced laterally due to the prostate gland. Had this CT been performed in the prone position it would be clearer that these stones are free in the bladder.

> If leukocytes remain positive but culture/nitrites are negative, this is likely to be due to residual inflammation but consider other causes of sterile pyuria (*Box 3.11*).

> In men with a UTI in adolescence, recurrent UTI, or a single episode of pyelonephritis or prostatitis, a urology review should be arranged.

> Recurrent UTI (defined as ≥2 MSU-proven UTIs within 6 months or ≥3 within 12 months) always warrants urological evaluation. There are numerous mechanisms to prevent recurrent UTIs, including counselling and behavioural modifications, non-antimicrobial prophylaxis and antimicrobial prophylaxis. Good stewardship of antibiotics is an important concept (*Box 3.12*). Antibiotic prophylaxis should not be prescribed without specialist input.

N.B.: up to 50% of those with 'UTI symptoms' will not have a proven UTI. Consider other causes of urinary symptoms (*Box 3.13*),

Box 3.11 Causes of sterile pyuria (≥10 white cells per high-power field ×400 without bacteria).

- Stones.
- Partially/recently treated UTI.
- Tuberculosis
- Carcinoma *in situ*.
- Schistosomiasis.
- Interstitial cystitis.

Box 3.12 Multi-resistant infection and antibiotic stewardship.

The lack of novel antimicrobials being developed and the increasing burden of resistant organisms is already becoming problematic in primary and secondary care. To address this growing problem, antimicrobial stewardship has become hugely important. The main principles are prescribing antibiotics only when needed (not for self-limiting infections) and regularly reviewing the ongoing requirement for them. Local antibiotic guidelines should be in place that will be influenced by local pathogen properties and should be closely adhered to.

Box 3.13 Non-infective causes of cystitis.

- Bladder pain syndrome/interstitial cystitis (more common in women).
- Radiation cystitis (following prostatic, rectal or gynaecological radiotherapy).
- Drug-induced cystitis (such as with cyclophosphamide).
- Urothelial carcinoma (particularly carcinoma *in situ* can cause irritative/storage urinary symptoms).

many of which will require urological investigation. Standard laboratory MC&S will report bacteriuria if a single organism is identified at a concentration of 10^5cfu/ml or higher. However, it is recognised that patients may have a UTI at lower counts which may not be picked up by the lab (false negatives). Maintain a high level of suspicion, and take into account the patient's history, examination, observations and inflammatory markers, particularly in patients who report a history of recurrent problems or cystitis. Consider discussion with microbiology colleagues for further advice.

Catheter-associated UTI

Indwelling urinary catheters significantly increase the risk of UTI, leading to a daily risk of UTI of between 5% and 7%. In hospital-acquired UTIs, 80% are due to catheters. Like any foreign body, catheters are quickly coated by a biofilm of bacteria. Given that catheters are invariably colonised, treatment with antibiotics is usually reserved only for those with symptomatic infection (e.g. suprapubic pain, pyrexia or offensive/turbid urine) or undergoing urological intervention. If a catheter has been in place for >7 days, it is advised that the catheter should be changed before or shortly after starting antibiotic treatment.

Key Points

- If patients are on the correct antibiotics but have persistent symptoms, consider reimaging to exclude an abscess or urinary tract obstruction.
- The judicious use, and appropriate duration, of antibiotics is vital in controlling antibiotic resistance.
- Be aware of other causes of UTI symptoms and refer if necessary, especially if there is any associated haematuria.
- Only treat symptomatic UTIs – to reduce the development of antibiotic-resistant organisms*.
- Consider the risk of sepsis in all patients with signs of infection.
- Dipstick urinalysis is a quick and useful investigative tool, but is not 100% sensitive for UTI.

*Exceptions include pregnancy and prior to invasive urological procedures.

PROSTATITIS[4]

Acute bacterial prostatitis

Acute bacterial prostatitis is new-onset bacterial infection of the prostate.

Acute bacterial prostatitis (**Figure 3.12**) can be thought of as a 'complicated UTI'. The majority of cases are thought to occur from infected urine refluxing into the prostatic ducts in the urethra. The prevalence is not as high as cystitis but increases through adulthood. Iatrogenic prostatitis has become the most common presentation, with transrectal prostate biopsy a higher risk than transperineal approaches. The spectrum of pathogens is similar to those in *Box 3.9*, page 60, with *E. coli* again the most common organism.

Multiple categories or 'types' of pro-statitis exist (*Box 3.14*). Chronic forms are a major cause of pelvic pain in men and can be very difficult to treat. Early recognition

and effective treatment of acute prostatitis can reduce this associated morbidity.

Presentation
- Systemically unwell with acute onset.
- Fever, nausea, vomiting.
- Pelvic, back, perineal or groin pain, or pain in the external genitalia are all seen.
- Voiding dysfunction (frequency, straining, weak flow, pain) +/- urinary retention.

Examination
- Pyrexia +/- signs of sepsis.
- Exquisitely tender +/- swollen prostate on DRE.
- Patients may have signs of associated urinary retention.

Investigation
- Urinalysis and culture.
- FBC, U&E, CRP, glucose, ABG if systemically unwell.
- Post-void bladder scan.
- Consider imaging (MRI/transrectal USS/CT) if there is a high suspicion of prostatic abscess.

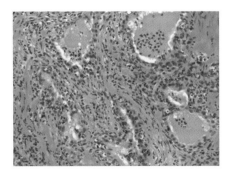

Figure 3.12 Microscopic image of acute prostatitis. A haematoxylin and eosin-stained section from a prostate biopsy showing collections of neutrophils within the gland lumina and also infiltrating the glandular epithelium and surrounding connective tissue. (Image courtesy of Dr Anne Warren.)

Box 3.14 Types of prostatitis.

- Type I: acute bacterial.
- Type II: chronic bacterial.
- Type IIIa: chronic pelvic pain syndrome (inflammatory).
- Type IIIb: chronic pelvic pain syndrome (non-inflammatory).
- Type IV: asymptomatic inflammatory (identified on prostate histology).

- Do NOT perform a PSA: this is not diagnostic, will be elevated and will NOT be helpful.

Management
- ABCDE approach (see page 185) and sepsis management (see page 12 or page 183).
- IV antibiotics as per local hospital guidelines: often gentamicin and a broad-spectrum agent such as co-amoxiclav or piperacillin/tazobactam.
- Analgesia.
- Prolonged course of oral antibiotics according to sensitivity (2–4 weeks) after acute phase. In chronic bacterial prostatitis, a 4–6-week course of oral antibiotics is commonly used.
- Avoid urethral catheterisation if possible (thought to prevent drainage and prolong infection), although this may be needed for acute urinary retention. An alternative is to insert a suprapubic catheter.
- If slow to improve consider a prostatic abscess (*Box 3.15* and **Figure 3.13**), which will require drainage either by the transurethral or transrectal route.

Box 3.15 Risk factors for prostatic abscess formation.

- *E. coli* prostatitis.
- Immunocompromised.
- Diabetes mellitus.
- Transurethral instrumentation/surgery.
- Urethral catheterisation.

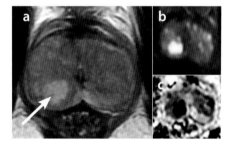

Figure 3.13 Magnetic resonance imaging showing a prostatic abscess. (**a**) Axial T2-weighted images with a focal high-signal abscess (arrow). A tumour would be seen as a low signal; (**b**) diffusion-weighted image and (**c**) apparent diffusion coefficient map indicating restricted diffusion in the abscess.

Key Points

- Consider a diagnosis of acute bacterial prostatitis in men presenting with systemic symptoms, a positive urine dipstick and recent prostate biopsy.
- Assess for and treat any associated urinary retention.
- Failure to respond to appropriate antibiotic treatment may suggest prostatic abscess formation.

URETHRITIS[5]

Urethritis is inflammation of the urethra; often with painful urination and purulent discharge.

The majority of urethritis is infective in origin. It can be broadly divided into gonococcal urethritis (*Neisseria gonorrhoeae*) and non-gonococcal urethritis (*Chlamydia trachomatis, Trichomonas vaginalis, Ureaplasma urealyticum, Mycoplasma genitalium*). These pathogens will often co-exist. Non-infective forms of urethritis include contact dermatitis (from soaps or spermicides used in the genital area), trauma and foreign objects in the urethra causing blood-stained discharge.

Reiter's syndrome refers to a reactive arthritis, often in association with urethritis and conjunctivitis. It is commonly triggered by chlamydial infection.

Presentation and examination

Gonorrhoea usually presents with a purulent urethral discharge, whereas non-gonococcal urethritis tends to present with a mucoid discharge. In men there may be erythema surrounding the urethral meatus. The foreskin should be retracted and urethral meatus examined to distinguish between discharge from under the prepuce (smegma, balanitis) and true urethral discharge. In women the disease may be asymptomatic. Rectal and pharyngeal gonorrhoea infection can occur in both sexes, but also tend to be asymptomatic.

Complications include epididymitis, urethral strictures, pelvic inflammatory disease and reduced fertility.

Investigation
- Superficial and deep urethral swabs.
- First-pass urine samples. Most tests rely on nucleic acid amplification testing.
- Urine samples often look turbid, if due to urethritis as opposed to UTI; this will clear on mid- or late-stream samples.

Management

Gonorrhoea is treated with either a single oral dose of cefixime 400mg or intramuscular dose of ceftriaxone 250mg. *Chlamydia trachomatis* is treated with a single oral dose of azithromycin (1g) or 7 days of oral doxycycline (100mg BD). Resistance to first-line therapies is rising in some areas and local guidelines should be followed. Fluoroquinolones (ciprofloxacin, ofloxacin) are usually effective against both pathogens, but are not usually first line.

Patients should be advised to attend a genito-urinary medicine (GUM) or sexual health clinic. They can arrange anonymous contact tracing. Sexual intercourse should be avoided until the patient and their partner have completed treatment.

Key Points
- Urethritis is often a sexually transmitted infection.
- Patients should be advised to attend a sexual health or genito-urinary medicine clinic. These clinics can arrange contact tracing if necessary.

References

1 Fisher E, Subramonian K, Omar MI. The role of alpha blockers prior to removal of urethral catheter for acute urinary retention in men. *Cochrane Database of Syst Rev* 2014; **6**. Art. No.: CD006744. DOI: 10.1002/14651858.CD006744.pub3.

2 Price SJ, Shephard EA, Stapley SA, *et al.* Non-visible versus visible haematuria and bladder cancer risk: a study of electronic records in primary care. *Br J Gen Pract* 2014; **64**: 584–9.

3 Khadra MH, Pichard RS, Charlton M, *et al.* A prospective analysis of 1930 patients with haematuria to evaluate current diagnostic practice. *J Urol* 2000; **163**: 524–7.

4 National Institute for Health and Care Excellence (NICE). Suspected Cancer: Recognition and Referral. NICE Guidance (NG12), June 2015. https://www.nice.org.uk/guidance.

5 Anderson J, Fawcett D, Feehally J, *et al.* Joint Consensus Statement on the Initial Assessment of Haematuria. On behalf of the Renal Association and British Association of Urological Surgeons. July 2008.

Chapter 4

Genitoscrotal Emergencies

Michal Sut and CJ Shukla

ACUTE SCROTUM

Acute scrotum is a general term referring to an emergency condition affecting the contents or the wall of the scrotum.

There are a number of conditions that present acutely, predominantly with pain and/or swelling (*Table 4.1*). A careful and detailed history and examination, and in some cases, investigations allow differentiation between these diagnoses. A prompt diagnosis is essential as the patient may require urgent surgical intervention.

Testicular torsion

Testicular torsion refers to twisting of the spermatic cord, causing ischaemia of the testicle.

Testicular torsion is a true emergency and an organ-threatening condition. 'Missed torsion' may have a significant impact on the patient (e.g. psychosexual, behavioural, hormonal, reproductive), as well as potentially on the clinician (medicolegal). Despite widespread awareness of the condition, the ability to differentiate testicular torsion from other scrotal emergencies could still be improved. Testicular ischaemia leads to irreversible loss of reproductive germinal tissue within

hours of onset. It is therefore of paramount importance to assess these patients without delay.

Pathophysiology

There is a bimodal distribution of testicular torsion with peak incidences in infants and again in young adolescents (age 7–15 years), although presentation can be at any age, including very rarely in men over 40. The pathophysiology is secondary to twisting/torsion of the spermatic cord within (intravaginal) or including (extravaginal torsion) the tunica vaginalis. Extravaginal torsion tends to occur in newborn boys and is much less common than intravaginal torsion. Torsion of the testis and spermatic cord results in impaired venous return, congestion and oedema, leading to reduced arterial blood flow, ischaemia and eventually infarction of testicular tissue.

History

At the initial assessment patients report a sudden onset of pain. The pain may wake them from sleep, or start after strenuous exercise, minor trauma to the genitals or sexual activity. In general, a gradual onset of pain is atypical for torsion and other diagnoses should be strongly considered.

Table 4.1 Differential diagnosis for acute scrotum.

Ischaemia	Testicular torsion Torsion of testicular appendage Testicular infarction
Infectious	Acute epididymitis Acute epididymo-orchitis Acute orchitis Fournier's gangrene Abscess
Hernia	Strangulated inguinoscrotal hernia, with or without associated testicular ischaemia
Acute on chronic conditions	Hydrocoele infection Testicular tumour with infection, bleeding or ischaemia Varicocoele
Trauma	Ruptured testicle Scrotal/testicular haematoma or haematocoele

Previous episodes of similar pain with spontaneous resolution is occasionally reported and may suggest intermittent testicular torsion. In this scenario, the testis torts and detorts without causing irreversible ischaemia. This group of patients are at risk of a progression to complete torsion and should have their testis fixed urgently.

A familial history of a father or brother with proven testicular torsion may be present, as an anatomical variant of a bell-clapper abnormality can be hereditary.

Examination
- Inspection: patients with testicular torsion are in significant pain that is worse on movement. This is particularly noticeable when the patient attempts to walk, often with a wide-based, slow gait. We suggest examination of the scrotum both in standing and lying positions. When the patient is upright, the affected testis is high-riding and may appear swollen. It is useful to confirm with the patient whether or not this is his normal anatomy. The overlying scrotal skin can be erythematous.
- Palpation: this is undertaken with the patient in the supine position. Typically, the testis is mildly enlarged but may feel firm and slightly irregular; this is the result of the aforementioned vascular engorgement. The torted testis is tender and the cord structures are often difficult/impossible to palpate. Patients may present much later, after several days, and at that stage the pain may have resolved due to testicular infarction.

Investigation

Diagnosis of testicular torsion is a clinical one and any tests should be done only under the proviso they do not delay surgical exploration in cases of suspected torsion. They are generally useful to confirm a suspected alternative diagnosis such as epididymo-orchitis. If there is diagnostic uncertainty, surgical exploration is the only infallible diagnostic test.

Doppler ultrasound may show absent blood flow to the testis but in cases of torsion with less than a 360° twist, some blood flow may still be apparent; therefore, ultrasound cannot be relied upon to accurately exclude a torsion.

Laboratory tests may be normal or report mild white cell count (WCC) and C-reactive protein (CRP) elevation corresponding with tissue ischaemia within the testis.

Management

Testicular torsion is managed with scrotal exploration and bilateral fixation of both testes if viable. In cases of an infarcted non-viable testis, this should be excised (orchidectomy) and the contralateral testis fixed (orchidopexy). Where there is questionable testicular viability, the testis should be detorted and wrapped in a warm saline-soaked swab for 15 minutes before re-evaluating.

If the attending doctor is concerned about testicular torsion, they should immediately notify the appropriate team (urology, paediatric surgery or general surgery) and start preparing the patient for theatre (ensure the patient is 'nil by mouth', check bloods, give intravenous [IV] fluids and analgesia).

Torsion of testicular appendage (torted hydatid of Morgagni)

This uncommon condition is a result of a twist of a vestigial remnant of the Müllerian duct or Wolffian duct (**Figure 4.1**) at the upper pole of the testis.

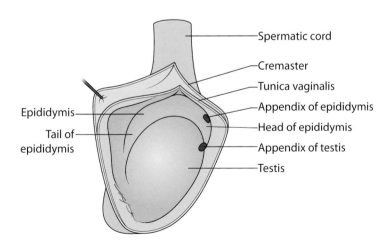

Spermatic cord

Cremaster

Tunica vaginalis

Appendix of epididymis

Head of epididymis

Appendix of testis

Testis

Epididymis

Tail of epididymis

Figure 4.1 The locations of the testicular appendages. The appendix testis is a remnant of the Müllerian duct, whereas the epididymal appendix is a remnant of the Wolffian duct.

History
- Pain also develops rapidly in a similar fashion to testicular torsion.
- The severity of pain is usually less; however, this is subjective and may not reliably distinguish between this and testicular torsion.
- Usually affects younger children (pre-pubertal), making the clinical history more difficult to obtain and somewhat less reliable.

Examination
- Inspection typically reveals a discoloured, ischaemic appendage of the testis which, in Caucasians, can be seen through thin scrotal skin as a 'blue dot sign' (**Figure 4.2**) associated with the upper pole of the testis.
- Palpation may be difficult, especially in younger patients, but if possible, then elicited tenderness is usually confined to the upper pole of the affected testis, rather than throughout the testis.

Investigation
As for testicular torsion.

Management
If there is any doubt about the diagnosis, scrotal exploration should be done to exclude testicular torsion. If a confident diagnosis can be made, conservative management with regular pain relief can be embarked upon. However, scrotal exploration and excision of the torted appendix should be considered as this will firstly confirm the diagnosis and, secondly, alleviate the pain more rapidly than expectant management.

Epididymo-orchitis

Epididymo-orchitis is an infective process affecting the testis (orchitis), epididymis (epididymitis) or both (epididymo-orchitis).

The aetiology varies between age groups. In young, sexually active men, sexually-transmitted infections (STIs) due to chlamydia or gonorrhoea are the most likely causes, while in older men ascending Gram-negative infections, predominantly with *Escherichia coli* from the urinary tract, on a background of poor bladder emptying is the more common cause. This is not absolute, and a detailed sexual history is still necessary. Rarely, and especially if appropriately-treated infection does not resolve and certain risk factors are present

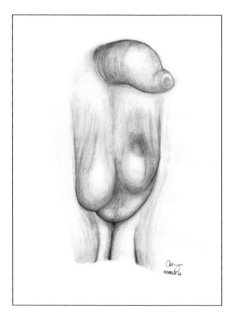

Figure 4.2 Blue dot sign. Torted hydatid of Morgagni of the left hemiscrotum. (Illustration by Dr O. Kenyon.)

(immunosuppression, travel to endemic areas, bacillus Calmette–Guérin [BCG] treatment for bladder cancer), tuberculosis-related epididymitis and orchitis should be excluded.

History
Gradually increasing pain and swelling of the hemiscrotum with or without associated fevers is typically reported. It is important to enquire about sexual behaviour, lower urinary tract symptoms (LUTS), previous episodes and risk factors for tuberculosis (TB) as this will guide appropriate management.

Examination
- Typically, the affected hemiscrotum looks markedly enlarged and erythematous, but changes may spread and involve the contralateral testis. It is crucial to inspect the entire scrotal skin, including the perineal aspect in order not to miss any areas of skin necrosis that may suggest the development of Fournier's gangrene (see page 88).
- Palpate and percuss the suprapubic area to assess for a distended urinary bladder.
- Rectal examination of the prostate looking for an enlarged gland due to benign prostatic enlargement (BPE) causing bladder outlet obstruction (BOO) and for prostatitis or prostatic abscess.

Investigation
- Record vital signs and in the case of hospital admission monitor patients on a regular basis, looking for any signs of systemic inflammatory response (SIRS) and to assess the response to treatment.
- WCC and CRP should be tested to assess severity of the infection.
- Urine dipstick may reveal a background urinary tract infection (UTI), in which case mid-stream urine (MSU) samples should be sent for culture and sensitivity. In younger patients (<35 years of age) or older patients with a risk of STIs, urinary polymerase chain reaction (PCR) tests for chlamydia and gonorrhoea tests are also necessary prior to treatment.
- A post-void residual (PVR) bladder scan to assess for adequate bladder emptying.
- Scrotal ultrasound scanning (USS) should be done acutely to exclude a collection or an abscess, or if there is any doubt about the diagnosis, e.g. tumour or missed torsion. A follow-up scan should also be considered to look for resolution of the changes and exclude underlying testicular malignancy that may present as an infective episode (**Figures 4.3, 4.4**).

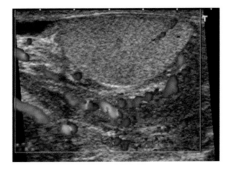

Figure 4.3 Colour Doppler ultrasound image showing a normal testicle with a thickened epididymis lying posteriorly, with increased vascularity in keeping with epididymitis.

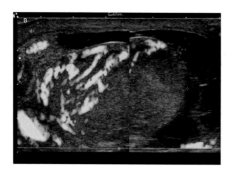

Figure 4.4 Longitudinal ultrasound image of the right testicle with power Doppler showing a heterogeneous testicle with significant increased vascularity and an adjacent loculated hydrocoele, in keeping with orchitis with a secondary hydrocoele.

Management

Antibiotics should be given orally or IV depending on the severity of infection. In the case of significant sepsis, aminoglycosides in the form of gentamicin could be combined with either broad-spectrum penicillins (e.g. co-amoxiclav) or fluoroquinolones (e.g. ciprofloxacin, ofloxacin).

Oral antibiotics are given empirically according to the most likely pathogenic organism and local policy. Therefore, young, sexually active men should be treated with fluoroquinolones with activity against *Chlamydia trachomatis* (e.g. ofloxacin or levofloxacin); alternatively, doxycycline 100mg twice-daily for two weeks. If a STI is not suspected, co-amoxiclav or ciprofloxacin could be given. In suspected TB, the infectious disease/microbiology team should be consulted.

A urinary catheter should be considered if bladder emptying is significantly affected (PVR >300ml). Any recurrent UTIs and LUTS should be managed accordingly in the outpatient setting after resolution of infection.

Scrotal abscess

A collection of pus within the deep layers of the scrotum is termed correctly as a scrotal abscess.

Not infrequently, superficial infections within hair follicles or primary perineal abscesses with some scrotal skin involvement are also labelled the same. The significance of a correct diagnosis relates to the fact that the latter should be managed by colorectal or general surgeons. Scrotal abscesses almost exclusively develop on the background of other infective conditions (e.g. epididymo-orchitis, UTI, urine extravasation due to urethral stricture disease).

History

Patients usually report gradually increasing swelling and pain that develop on the background of another condition, usually epididymo-orchitis. Febrile episodes related to SIRS are not uncommon, and like other abscesses there may be swinging fevers. Patient-related risk factors include diabetes mellitus, immunodeficiency and poor bladder emptying.

Examination

Generalised swelling and tenderness associated with erythema can be seen on the ipsilateral side. Commonly, fluctuance can be palpated over the area where the collection is nearest to scrotal skin. It is very important to exclude the presence of necrotising infection by carefully inspecting the skin for any signs of necrosis or skin crepitus. The testis is usually easily palpable and may be found lying normally in the scrotum but is commonly irregular and warm due to the underlying infection.

Investigation
- Inflammatory markers (WCC, CRP) are commonly elevated.
- Scrotal USS confirms an underlying collection, which may have characteristics of purulent fluid and may also identify underlying pathology (**Figure 4.5**).

Management
Immediate management constitutes broad-spectrum antibiotic cover. Fluid resuscitation and pain relief should be considered and bladder catheterisation might be required if PVR volumes are high.

In most cases, surgical exploration and drainage of the abscess is indicated. A trial of conservative management may be an option in selected cases presenting early with small abscesses and no clinical signs of septicaemia. However, this is only acceptable as an inpatient where regular re-examination of the scrotum is done and vital signs as well as inflammatory markers are monitored. In such cases, progression or lack of improvement requires surgical exploration and drainage of the collection. In cases of associated skin necrosis or suspected Fournier's gangrene, the overlying skin and superficial fascia may also require debridement (see page 88). Orchidectomy is rarely required.

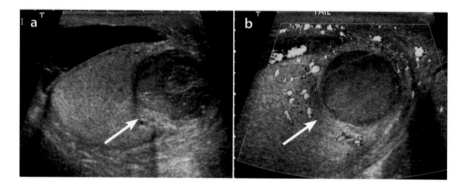

Figure 4.5 Ultrasound images of the testicle in grey scale (**a**) and power Doppler (**b**) showing a well-defined hypoechoic avascular testicular abscess (arrow).

Hydrocoele/infected hydrocoele

A hydrocoele is an abnormal accumulation of serous fluid around a testicle, also termed a 'hydrocoele testis'.

The space between the tunica albuginea casing of the testis and its surrounding fascia is physiologically filled with a small amount of yellow straw fluid within the tunica vaginalis, a coelomic sac derivative, which allows smooth traction between both surfaces. As a result of some insult (e.g. minor trauma, infection), the amount of fluid can increase significantly. It can in rare circumstances present acutely, either as a result of infection within a pre-existing hydrocoele, or as an acute hydrocoele secondary to epididymo-orchitis.

History

Due to the pathophysiological mechanisms explained above, presentation may be related to a new onset of scrotal swelling or infection of a chronic swelling. In the first scenario, symptoms of epididymo-orchitis may be present or minor trauma may be reported by the patient. Alternatively, patients may complain of an asymptomatic hydrocoele increasing in size, becoming tender or warm, which may or may not be associated with systemic upset.

Examination

Hemi-scrotal swelling should be smooth and fluctuant to varying degrees depending on the pressure within the sac. It is possible to palpate above the swelling, which differentiates it from an inguinoscrotal hernia. In a case of infected hydrocoele the hemi-scrotum may feel warm and tender. Typically the swelling transilluminates when a pen-torch light

is applied, although this sign may be lost due to turbidity of infected hydrocoele fluid. The testis is often not palpable as a separate entity to the fluid swelling.

Investigation

- Inflammatory markers in the form of WCC and CRP should be checked if an infection is suspected.
- USS of the scrotum is utilised to differentiate between a simple hydrocoele, infected hydrocoele and scrotal abscess. It may also report underlying epididymo-orchitis. Fluid turbidity and the presence of septations is usually noted in an infected hydrocoele as opposed to a simple hydrocoele (**Figure 4.6**).

Management

A reactive hydrocoele is not a true emergency and is not treated as such. Treatment of underlying epididymo-orchitis might alleviate the size of the swelling. Alternatively, elective repair of the hydrocoele may be performed.

An infected hydrocoele may be treated conservatively with either oral or IV antibiotics according to the severity of infection. Broad-spectrum antibiotics in the form of co-amoxiclav or fluoroquinolones (e.g. ciprofloxacin, ofloxacin) can be administered orally (also, see local microbiology guidelines). In cases of more severe infection, for any of the above conditions, antibiotics may be used IV with the addition of gentamicin, according to hospital guidelines.

If an infected hydrocoele fails to respond to conservative treatment, or in severe infections with systemic upset, drainage in the operating theatre is indicated. Patients

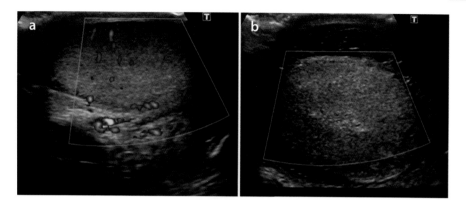

Figure 4.6 Power Doppler ultrasound images showing normal vascularity in the right testicle (**a**) and infarcted left testicle (**b**). The left testis is enlarged and heterogeneous with no blood flow and a surrounding echogenic loculated hydrocoele.

should be counselled on the possibility of an orchidectomy if the underlying testis has necrosed from an abscess.

Scrotal haematoma

A scrotal haematoma is a collection of blood within the scrotum.

This may be secondary to trauma, or iatrogenic as a result of elective procedures such as hydrocoele repair or vasectomy. Blood may collect in specific anatomic layers and this will determine the necessity for treatment and outcomes. Blood may collect within the tunica vaginalis, known as a haematocoele (this is where hydrocoele fluid accumulates), between the testis and scrotal wall (following hydrocoele surgery) or within the muscular layers of the scrotal wall.

History

The patient may report a previous direct blow to the genital area or a recent scrotal surgical procedure. Spontaneous bleeding happens very rarely, although it can present in the age extremes in relation to systemic diseases (e.g. Henoch–Schönlein purpura, bleeding diathesis) or anticoagulation (warfarin), which can be elicited during history taking.

Examination

The hemi-scrotum is usually uniformly enlarged, bruised and depending on the size of the haematoma, might be tense. The swelling is typically mildly tender, and in cases of infected collection it may be warm. Severe tenderness is usually due to an underlying pathology, e.g. testis rupture from trauma, infection, etc.

Investigation

Laboratory tests including FBC, CRP and clotting screen should be done in the first instance. Although extremely unlikely, checking haemoglobin (Hb) will confirm whether blood loss is significant. If there is a significant drop in Hb, suspect blood loss from the operation (on table) or post-operatively (e.g. bleeding from the testicular artery which can retract into the abdomen following an inguinal orchidectomy). In cases of infected haematoma, one would expect an elevated WCC and CRP. A clotting screen will be deranged in haematological diseases.

Scrotal USS is the examination of choice to confirm the presence of echodense fluid in the scrotum. The role of USS is also to rule out features of infection as well as assessing testicular integrity in trauma cases.

Management

- Most commonly, conservative management is sufficient with prophylactic oral antibiotics to prevent infection. Co-amoxiclav for 7–10 days is appropriate. Even minor haematomas take weeks to reabsorb and the patient should be advised of this on discharge. More significant haematomas causing pain/discomfort from the distension can be drained surgically.

- In cases of trauma leading to testicular injury, or signs of infected haematoma, scrotal exploration should be undertaken as an emergency procedure.

- Any spontaneous bleeding related to an underlying systemic disorder should have the background problem addressed by the appropriate team.

Key Points

- Testicular torsion is a urological emergency.

- Suspected torsion should be assessed rapidly as patients should reach the operating theatre within 6 hours of symptom onset.

- Previous episodes of similar short-lived pain and a family history of proven testicular torsion may be reported in the history.

- Sudden onset and significant testicular pain are usually present; consider an alternative diagnosis otherwise.

- The typical examination findings of torsion is a unilateral high-riding and swollen testis, tender to palpation throughout.

- With the exception of suspected torsion (when exploration should not be delayed), ultrasound is the investigation of choice for most scrotal pathology.

PENILE EMERGENCIES

This topic will cover the acute presentations of penile fracture, paraphimosis and balanitis in the emergency setting. Priapism will be covered separately on pages 84–87.

Penile fracture

A penile fracture is a rupture in the tunica albuginea of the penis.

This uncommon injury occurs due to trauma to the erect penis, usually during sexual intercourse. During a rigid erection, the engorged corpora cavernosa are contained by the fibrous layer of the tunica albuginea. The thickness of tunica wall usually measures around 2mm but when the penis is erect it is stretched to about only 0.25mm, which affects its tensile strength. If a strong bending force is applied in this situation, it can lead to rupture of the tunical layer (usually at the ventrolateral aspect).

History

Taking a clear history is vital for achieving the correct diagnosis (*Box 4.1*). Most men report sudden pain, an audible sound ('snap', 'pop' or 'crack') and immediate detumescence. In the majority of cases it is not possible to obtain an erection following the injury, although some patients with minor subtunical tears may retain some erectile capacity. For medicolegal purposes it is important that a baseline sexual function is established at the initial history, as erectile dysfunction (ED) is one of the recognised complications, especially if the presentation or treatment is delayed significantly (*Box 4.2*). A concomitant urethral injury occurs in approximately 10% (**Figure 4.7**) of cases and is often manifest by urethral bleeding or haematuria. In rare cases it may lead to the inability to void.

Box 4.1 Typical history of penile fracture.

- Mechanism of injury: bending force upon an erect penis.
- Audible sound ('pop', 'snap', 'crack') may or may not be present.
- Immediate/rapid detumescence.
- Subsequent inability to obtain an erection.
- Pain.

Box 4.2 Medicolegal advice in assessing a patient with penile fracture.

- Document the time since the injury and the man's baseline erectile function.
- Document any history of blood at the urethral meatus or haematuria.

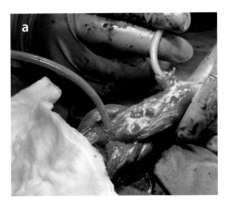
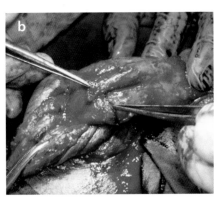

Figure 4.7 Intra-operative images from exploratory surgery in a male patient with penile fracture (**a** and **b**) demonstrating complete urethral disruption (**a**). Defects in both the corpora and urethra have been repaired (**b**). (Images by Jagodič K, *et al*, used under the Creative Commons Attribution licence 2.0 [http://creativecommons.org/licenses/by/2.0]. Jagodič K, Erklavec M, Bizjak I, *et al*. A case of penile fracture with complete urethral disruption during sexual intercourse: a case report. *Journal of Medical Case Reports* 2007; 1: 14. DOI: 10.1186/1752-1947-1-14.)

Examination

The classical 'aubergine sign' (**Figure 4.8**) is a typical clinical finding where there is tunical disruption with intact Buck's fascia. Although less dramatic, haematoma or bruising can occur due to the containment of the haematoma within the various penile tissue layers. A defect in the tunica albuginea may be palpable, most commonly in the area of most severe bruising, but tends to be easier to palpate in the operating theatre when the patient is anaesthetised. Differential diagnoses include injury to the superficial dorsal vein or suspensory ligament of the penis.

Investigation

- Penile fracture is a clinical diagnosis in the majority of cases, but in difficult situations, magnetic resonance imaging (MRI) or USS might be required to confirm the diagnosis.
- If urethral trauma is suspected, a urethrogram or cystoscopy can be performed to determine urethral integrity.

Management

- The treatment of choice is surgical repair and this should ideally be performed in the first 24–36 hours,

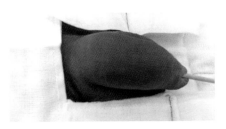

Figure 4.8 A patient about to undergo surgical exploration and repair of a suspected penile fracture exhibits the classical 'aubergine sign'.

although more recent studies confirm that surgical correction may be delayed beyond this if necessary (if patients present later). Surgical exploration is performed in order to evacuate the haematoma and repair the tunica albuginea, to prevent complications that include ED, penile curvature from fibrosis and pain.

- A gentle attempt at catheterisation in the case of associated urinary retention by an experienced team member or urologist is acceptable even in the event of blood in the meatus. However, in the case of failure, cystoscopy at the time of the repair may be required.

Paraphimosis

Paraphimosis refers to the inability to pull forward a retracted foreskin over the glans penis.

In healthy adults, a normal foreskin (prepuce) should allow easy retraction and reduction in both the flaccid and erect states. Some conditions may alter the anatomy of the prepuce or glans penis leading to a difficulty in retraction of the preputial opening over the glans penis.

These include a physiological phimosis or a pathological phimosis caused by balanitis xerotica obliterans (BXO) (*Table 4.2*). In these circumstances a retracted foreskin, especially in the erect penis or due to prolonged exposure (e.g. iatrogenic – following catheter placement), may result in a constricting band lying proximal to the glans. This leads to painful vascular engorgement/oedema of the glans, and more commonly oedema of the prepuce distal to the constricting band of tissue (**Figure 4.9**).

Presentation

Patients usually present with pain and swelling of the glans penis or distal prepuce but in some men, especially if elderly and confused, the condition might be reported by a carer or health care professional helping with personal hygiene. It is common in catheterised patients as manipulation of the prepuce increases the risk. Patients may have repetitive presentations if the underlying pathology has not been addressed.

Table 4.2 Risk factors for paraphimosis.

Phimosis/tight foreskin
Indwelling catheter
Poor hygiene
Carer dependence
(All associated with a failure to replace the foreskin correctly)

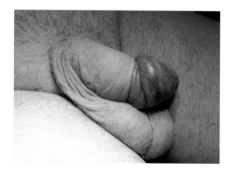

Figure 4.9 Paraphimosis in a 45-year-old diabetic patient. (Image by Drvgaikwad used under the Creative Commons licence 3.0 (http://creativecommons.org/licenses/by/3.0), via Wikimedia Commons. Image cropped by authors.)

Although very uncommon, an untreated tight paraphimosis can lead to ischaemic necrosis of the glans and preputial skin, and may potentially lead to fulminant infection of the genital skin (Fournier's gangrene). Therefore, any area of skin necrosis should be identified and debrided immediately.

Management

The immediate management of paraphimosis is to reduce it in a timely fashion, by replacing the narrow, constricting band of preputial tissue distal to the widest part of the glans, allowing vascular drainage and the oedema to subside. Rapid recognition of the condition and a prompt attempt at reduction increases the likelihood of success. Delayed presentation or recognition leads to worsening vascular engorgement and oedema that increases the requirement for surgical management under general anaesthesia.

In adults, a penile block can be used prior to reduction using a mixture of 10ml of 0.5% chirocaine and 10ml of 1% lidocaine (WITHOUT adrenaline) (see Chapter 7, page 166). General anaesthesia is usually more appropriate in the paediatric population.

Attempts to decrease the preputial swelling prior to reduction have been described, including ice packs or sugar application to the area (for an osmotic effect). Multiple orange needle punctures and then squeezing the oedematous fluid out of the tissue is another option known as the Dundee technique. The method preferred by the authors is a firm and increasing pressure on the glans penis to express the blood and oedema in order to decrease the swelling of the glans penis. The pressure applied is constant for a period of 5–10 minutes. Subsequently, an attempt at reduction of the tight foreskin over the less engorged glans penis is more likely to be successful. Rather than 'pulling' the foreskin over the glans it may be helpful to consider the procedure as 'pushing' the glans back through the tight foreskin. Some lubricant in the form of an aqueous jelly applied between the glans and prepuce can be helpful.

If manual reduction fails, involvement of the urologist is necessary on an urgent basis as a 'dorsal slit' or, very occasionally, emergency circumcision may be required. These are best done in an operating theatre environment.

After successful reduction, it is important to confirm that it is complete by palpating to ensure that the original constricting band lies distal to the glans, otherwise the patient will present again quickly with the same issue. Delayed definitive management, in the form of a circumcision, should be considered. The patient should therefore be referred for a urology opinion.

Balanitis

Balanitis is an inflammatory condition affecting the glans penis and occasionally also the inner lining of the prepuce (balanoposthitis).

Balanitis predominantly affects un-circumcised men and may cause an itch, soreness and redness of the skin leading to dysuria and discomfort in more severe cases. It can be non-infective (non-specific dermatitis, contact dermatitis) or infective (candidal, streptococcal, STI).

Diagnosis

Erythematous change to the skin covering the glans and/or prepuce and an associated itch or soreness are most frequently reported. If the affected area is very localised, contact dermatitis should be suspected. Streptococcal infections are usually associated with purulent exudate while candidal infections present with white creamy discolouration that may be easily wiped away.

Management

- It is important to be aware that penile cancer can resemble infection of the glans penis and therefore any suspicion of it should prompt consideration of penile biopsy.
- Most mild cases respond to con–servative measures such as daily cleaning with water or non-perfumed soap and using an emulsifying emollient, combined with the app–lication of a mild topical steroid cream for 1 week (such as hydrocortisone 1%) for one week, with the addition of an anti-fungal (imidazole cream).

- Early review after 2 weeks should be organized to assess the response to treatment and to ensure a cancer diagnosis is not missed.
- If symptoms do not resolve or are severe and recurrent, and underlying penile cancer is not suspected, a sub-preputial swab may help to isolate a causative organism to target therapy. Streptococcal balanitis is usually treated with flucloxacillin (500mg QDS) for 1 week or erythromycin (500mg QDS) or claryithromycin (250mg BD) in cases of penicillin allergy (refer to local microbiology guidelines).
- STI clinic referral should be considered in cases where a suspicion of sexually-derived infection exists.

Key Points

- Penile fracture has a classical history of pain, a 'snap' sound, and immediate detumescence.
- Early surgical repair is the mainstay of treatment for penile fracture.
- Prompt recognition and immediate reduction of paraphimosis is important.
- Surgical intervention is rarely required to reduce paraphimosis but delayed definitive management with circumcision should be considered.
- Be aware that penile cancer can sometimes resemble infection of the glans penis.

PRIAPISM

Priapism is an unwanted erection lasting over 4 hours, in the absence of sexual stimulation. The condition is named after Priapus, the Greek God of fertility.

Types of priapism
- Low-flow (ischaemic) accounts for 85%.
- Recurrent ischaemic priapism (also known as stuttering priapism).
- High-flow (non-ischaemic).

Ischaemic and stuttering priapism are urological emergencies. Irreversible ischaemic changes occur if the erection is prolonged for 4 hours, leading to ischaemic necrosis of the underlying erectile smooth muscle and resulting in a risk of permanent ED.

Presentation (see *Table 4.3*)
Ischaemic priapism behaves as a compartment syndrome of the penis. Due to the lack of venous outflow, the penis is extremely rigid and tender, and the patient presents with a painful erection. Typically, the corpus spongiosum is not involved and the glans is not rigid.

Stuttering priapism is a variant of ischaemic priapism with recurrent short-lived episodes of painful ischaemic priapic episodes lasting up to 2–3 hours, followed by spontaneous detumescence. This is most commonly seen in sickle cell disease patients. It can be a prelude to a 'full-blown' ischaemic priapic episode, and hence the need for urgent referral to an urologist.

Non-ischaemic priapism usually occurs after a history of a traumatic injury resulting in the formation of an arteriocavernous fistula (a fistula between one of the penile or bulbar arteries and the erectile cavernosal spaces). The most common mechanism is a blunt perineal injury. In this situation, as arterial blood is supplying the cavernous spaces with oxygenated blood, the patient has less pain in the penis itself and the management of this can be by observation initially, followed by arteriography and embolisation if necessary. In this situation, the patient has less rigidity of erection as the venous outflow channels are patent and hence the erection is 'compressible'. Non-ischaemic and stuttering priapism do require close follow-up as both can eventually manifest as an acute ischaemic

Table 4.3 Types of priapism and typical clinical findings.

	Low-flow	High-flow	Stuttering
Pain	Present	Absent/little	Present
Rigidity	Rigid	Semi-rigid	Rigid
Duration	>4h	>4h	2–3h
Aspirated blood	Dark (venous)	Bright (arterial)	Aspiration not indicated

priapism later. Non-ischaemic priapism can also become an ischaemic priapism in the long term.

Causes

Priapism is most commonly idiopathic but it may be related to multiple medical conditions, most commonly sickle cell disease, pelvic malignancy, spinal cord compression, trauma and drugs (*Table 4.4*).

History

- The patient reports a prolonged erection associated with or without pain.
- It is important to elicit a thorough medical history including other comorbidities (e.g. haemoglobinopathies, especially sickle cell disease), previous episodes, baseline erectile function including any treatment.

Table 4.4 Causes of priapism.

Haematological	Sickle cell disease Leukaemia Thalassemia Haemophilia
Traumatic	Penile trauma Perineal trauma Pelvic trauma Spinal cord injury
Neoplastic	Pelvic malignancy, metastatic disease (also known as malignant priapism) Penile cancer Lymphoma Myeloma Paraneoplastic syndrome
Pharmacological	Phosphodiesterase type 5 inhibitors (sildenafil, tadalafil, vardenafill) Intracavernosal injections (papaverine, prostaglandin E) Antidepressants (fluoxetine) Antipsychotics (risperidone, olanzapine) Anticoagulants (warfarin, heparin) Alcohol Recreational drugs (cocaine, cannabis)
Neurological	Prolapsed intervertebral disc Spinal tumour Multiple sclerosis
Toxic	Venom (scorpions, spiders) Prostatitis Syphilis Malaria

- Drug history including recreational drugs (e.g. cocaine, amphetamines) and the use of medication for the treatment of ED, particularly injectable prostaglandins.

Examination

On examination there is an erect penis with sparing of the glans penis (rigid corpora cavernosa with a flaccid corpus spongiosum).

Investigation

- FBC to look for any obvious signs of infection and haematological abnormality.
- Haemoglobinopathy screen to exclude sickle cell disease where clinically indicated.

Management

Low-flow (ischaemic) priapism

Within 2–6 hours of onset, attempt to create detumescence using an oral alpha-agonist treatment (e.g. pseudoephedrine cold remedies) to vasoconstrict arterial inflow. Advise vigorous exercise of lower limb muscles (e.g. advise the patient to run up a flight of stairs or vigorous cycling); this stimulates β3 adrenergic nerves and diverts blood away from the penis. If these measures are unsuccessful within 30 minutes of presentation, or in cases of prolonged erection (>4 hours), then emergency referral to a urologist is recommended.

The next step is to aspirate blood from the corpora cavernosa for both diagnostic and therapeutic reasons. This can be performed, following a local anaesthetic penile block, using a large-bore needle (often a venflon or butterfly needle) inserted either laterally at the base of the penis or through the glans, into one of the corpora cavernosa. The blood taken should be analysed in a blood gas machine. In low-flow (ischaemic) priapism, the blood being venous, is usually congealed, dark and deoxygenated in appearance. Typical blood gas values are a low pH, low oxygen and high carbon dioxide levels (*Table 4.5*).

If low-flow priapism is confirmed, therapeutic aspiration should be performed. Using the same needle, aspirate 50–100ml of blood from the corpora cavernosa. Aspiration in these cases is often difficult

Table 4.5 Blood gas testing parameters in ischaemic and non-ischaemic priapism compared to the normal flaccid penis.

Pathology	PO_2	PCO_2	pH
Normal/flaccid penis	40mmHg (5.3kPa)	50mmHg (6.6kPa)	7.35
Ischaemic priapism	<30mmHg (4kPa)	>60mmHg (8kPa)	<7.25
Non-ischaemic priapism	>90mmHg (12kPa)	<40mmHg (5.3kPa)	7.4

as the venous, poorly oxygenated blood is usually congealed within the cavernosal sinuses. However, if successful, the ideal outcome is to ultimately see bright red blood accompanying detumescence, which signifies reperfusion of the corpora with oxygenated arterial blood. If the penis remains detumescent, the patient can be admitted for observation in order to check for recurrence and the need for further treatment. It may be helpful to flush the corpora with sterile saline instilled through a cannula in the contralateral corpora in order to try to clear the thick, congealed blood.

If this fails, the next step in the treatment algorithm is injection of a sympathomimetic agent directly into the penile corpora, e.g. phenylephrine, adrenaline or metaraminol, into the cavernosal spaces through a wide-gauge needle (check exact doses in your national drug formulary). It is extremely important to monitor the patient's blood pressure and heart rate during administration, as both could increase precipitously. It is therefore best performed in the 'resuscitation room' with continuous cardiac monitoring.

If this fails, shunt procedures may be used to create a fistula between the corpora cavernosa and corpus spongiosum (or saphenous vein), in order to allow drainage via an alternative route. These procedures are performed under general anaesthesia. Techniques include distal shunts (e.g. Winter, Ebbehoj, T-Shunt, Al-Ghorab) and more proximal shunts (e.g. Quackels, Grayhack). Most would recommend discussion with a tertiary referral centre where decisions regarding primary insertion of a penile prosthesis may be taken for cases of prolonged ischaemia (>48–72 hours' duration), as well as cases requiring more proximal shunts as these procedures have a considerable risk of ED.

Stuttering priapism

Treat any prolonged ischaemic episodes as above. Involve haematology early, be aware of a possible sickle cell crisis and resuscitate accordingly. Oral alpha-agonist treatment, e.g. pseudoephedrine or etilefrine, are often prescribed in the acute setting.

Non-ischaemic (high-flow) priapism

- This condition is non-urgent and conservative management initially is acceptable.
- Further investigation with arteriography should be organised to identify the presence of a vascular fistula, which can then be treated with selective embolisation.

Key Points

- Identify ischaemic (low-flow) priapism urgently in those with a prolonged unwanted erection.
- FBC and sickle cell status should be checked in appropriate groups.
- Diagnostic aspiration can be followed by therapeutic aspiration and washout via a large-bore needle.
- Urology involvement and an andrology opinion should be sought.

FOURNIER'S GANGRENE

Fournier's gangrene is a fulminant and destructive inflammation of the genital and/or perineal area; a form of necrotising infection.

Initially described in the 18th Century, this condition was named after the French physician, Jean Alfred Fournier, who presented a series of cases of necrotising fasciitis of the genitalia and perineum. Despite advances in diagnostic pathways and antimicrobial treatments, Fournier's gangrene still carries a significant risk of severe morbidity and a mortality rate of at least 20–30%. Interestingly, of the five patients initially described by Fournier, every one survived!

Pathophysiology

The pathophysiological mechanism of this rapidly progressive condition involves an advancing area of microthrombotic necrosis caused by suppurative infection by polymicrobial flora. There are typically multiple organisms cultured from the infection site, which include aerobes (e.g. *E. coli*, *Klebsiella*, streptococci, staphylococci) and anaerobes (e.g. *Clostridia*) acting synergistically, as well as fungi (e.g. *Candida*) in some cases. Infection follows the fascial tissue planes of the perineal and genitoscrotal region and may extend into the buttocks and anterior abdominal wall. Usually the testes and cord structures in men are spared by virtue of their separate fascial compartment and isolated blood supply (**Figure 4.10**).

Prompt recognition of this condition, especially in the out-of-hospital setting, is of utmost importance, as failure to act immediately may lead to severe sepsis and multi-organ failure. This is demonstrated by the increased mortality observed in patients admitted to hospital with signs of SIRS. A severity score based on measurable variables at the time of hospital admission has been developed to assess prognosis (*Table 4.6*).[1]

History

The organisms responsible for the development of Fournier's gangrene gain entry to the genitoscrotal area via one or more of three portals: skin, genitalia or colorectal route (*Table 4.7*). A clinical history including the risk factors (*Table 4.8*) is essential to identify potential cases of Fournier's gangrene. These include poor skin quality and decreased sensation especially in combination with immobility, incontinence, recent surgery and immuno-suppression, e.g. from poorly-controlled diabetes.

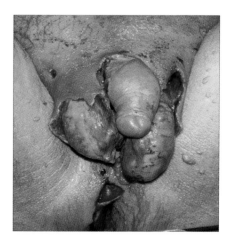

Figure 4.10 Fournier's gangrene after partial debridement. (Image used with permission of Elsevier Ltd. Bullock N, Doble A, Turner W, Cuckow P. *Urology: An Illustrated Colour Text.* Elsevier, Churchill Livingstone, 2007; p138, Fig. 1.)

Table 4.6 Fournier's Gangrene Severity Index.[1]

Physiological variables	High abnormal values				Normal values		Low abnormal values		
Assigned numerical score	4+	3+	2+	1+	0	1+	2+	3+	4+
Temperature (°C)	>41	39–40.9	-	38.5–38.9	36–38.4	34–35.9	32–33.9	30–31.9	<29.9
Heart rate (bpm)	>180	140–179	110–139	-	70–109	-	55–59	40–54	<39
Respiratory rate (bpm)	>50	35–49	-	25–34	12–24	10–11	6–9	-	<5
Serum sodium (mmol/L)	>180	160–179	155–159	150–154	130–149	-	120–129	111–119	<110
Serum potassium (mmol/L)	>7	6–6.9	-	5.5–5.4	3.5–4	3–3.4	2.5–2.9	-	<2.5
Serum creatinine (mg/100ml)	>3	2–3.4	1.5–1.9	-	0.6–1.4	-	<0.6	-	-
Hematocrit (%)	>60	-	50–59.9	46–49	30–45.9	-	20-29.9	-	<20
Leukocytes (total/mm³ × 1000)	>40	-	20–39.9	15–19.9	3–14.9	-	-	1–2.9	<1
Serum bicarbonate (mmol/L)	>52	41–51.9	-	32–40.9	22–31.9	-	18–21.9	15–17.9	<15

A deviation from normal is scored 1–4 according to the table from the original article. If the score is <9, the probability of survival is 78%; if ≥9, then the risk of death is 75%.

Table 4.7 Causes of Fournier's gangrene.

Skin	Genitalia	Colorectal
Perineal trauma Genital piercing Hydrocoele aspiration Vasectomy	Scrotal abscess Catheterisation Urethral stricture Prostatic biopsy Coital injury Infected Bartholin's gland Infected penile prosthesis Infected artificial urinary sphincter Incontinence tape/mesh procedure	Perianal abscess Rectal biopsy Anal dilatation Appendicitis Diverticulitis

Table 4.8 Pre-disposing factors for Fournier's gangrene.

Risk factors
Obesity
Diabetes
Immunodeficiency (immunosuppression, human immunodeficiency virus, leukaemia, etc.)
Alcohol abuse
Steroid use
Liver disease
Decreased mobility
Poor hygiene

Examination

It is paramount to have a high index of suspicion when assessing all patients with genitoscrotal infection. Every area of the skin and perineum should be carefully inspected and palpated. This may be challenging, especially in elderly patients and in those with poor mobility. However, there should be no compromise in evaluating these patients who are at particular risk of pressure sores that can predispose to Fournier's gangrene.

During examination it is vital to exclude any area of necrosis. These are usually easy to recognise as distinct black areas on the skin. Less advanced cases may present with severe spreading erythema with crepitus within the skin due to the presence of gas-forming organisms. There is often an associated offensive putrid smell. Severe tenderness that seems disproportionate, and SIRS in the presence of skin changes in the genitoscrotal region should also be treated with suspicion. The diagnosis is usually made clinically; however, if the diagnosis is uncertain, imaging can play a role. Computed tomography can demonstrate subcutaneous gas and tissue inflammation (**Figure 4.11**).

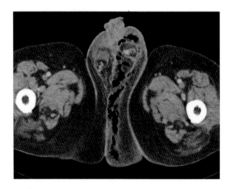

Figure 4.11 Axial computed tomography image showing extensive subcutaneous gas, and mild adjacent inflammatory change in the left perineum and scrotum. Surgical emphysema is a late sign of Fournier's gangrene.

Management

Fournier's gangrene should be treated with urgent surgical debridement of the affected areas down to healthy tissue. If there is any doubt regarding the diagnosis (e.g. suspected severe cellulitis), it is imperative to consult a specialist and a multi-disciplinary approach is usually best. It is useful to mark any involved areas for future comparison; these should be checked regularly, preferably by the same individual. Where there is evidence of progression, immediate surgical intervention may be necessary.

The key principles in the management of Fournier's gangrene are prompt recognition and a multi-disciplinary approach. Haemodynamic stability may not be achieved by fluid resuscitation alone and early involvement of the intensive care team to assist with inotropic and multiorgan support is advised. After obtaining blood samples for microbiological cultures at presentation, broad-spectrum antimicrobial therapy guided by local protocols should be started urgently, and usually consists of antibiotics to cover both aerobes and anaerobes (and occasionally fungal infections). Depending on local hospital policy and expertise, but also on the extent of the area affected and its pathology, several different surgical specialties may be involved in the care of these patients, including urological, colorectal and plastic surgeons.

The principle behind surgical management is to debride the necrotic area down to healthy, well-vascularised and well-oxygenated tissue. Surgical debridement most commonly needs to be repeated after 24 hours and sometimes on multiple occasions thereafter. This should be performed until the surgeon is satisfied that the residual tissue margins are healthy, bleeding and not involved by the disease process. Sometimes a suprapubic catheter is helpful to divert urine and bowel defunctioning may be required. Plastic surgeons play an important role in reconstructive procedures after the infection has been overcome, utilising techniques including skin flaps and grafts. Recovery may be lengthy and involve rehabilitation and counselling due to body image changes following extensive skin debridement.

Key Points

Multi-modal approach to Fournier's management:

- A high index of suspicion in patients with genital/perineal infection considering recognised risk factors.

- Resuscitation: urgent involvement of the necessary teams including surgeons and intensive care physicians for restoration of haemodynamic stability and multi-organ support.

- Antimicrobial therapy: broad-spectrum antibiotics covering aerobes, anaerobes and fungi.

- Surgical debridement: principal component of treatment. Several visits to the operating theatre might be required.

References

1   Laor E, Palmer TS, Tolia BM, *et al*. Outcome prediction in patients with Fournier's gangrene. *J Urol* 1995; **154**: 89–92.

Chapter 5

Trauma in Urology

Tom Mitchell and James Armitage

Urological trauma may be classified into that affecting the upper urinary tract; the lower urinary tract; and genitoscrotal trauma *(Box 5.1)*.

UPPER URINARY TRACT TRAUMA

Upper urinary tract trauma encompasses trauma to the kidneys and ureters.

Causes

Renal trauma occurs in approximately 3% of all trauma cases and 10% of those with abdominal trauma. There is a 3:1 male to female predominance, reflecting overall trends in trauma exposure. Of patients with renal trauma, there is a 40% incidence of other associated intra-abdominal injuries (rising to 80% if the aetiology of the injury was penetrating).

In the developed world, the majority of traumatic ureteric injuries are iatrogenic, from pelvic cancer surgery, gynaecological surgery, abdominal surgery or ureteroscopy.

Presentation

Blunt trauma accounts for the majority of renal injuries. Two mechanisms of injury may occur: direct trauma may crush the

Box 5.1 Classification of urological trauma.

- Upper urinary tract: renal and ureteric trauma.
- Lower urinary tract: bladder and urethral trauma.
- Genitoscrotal: trauma to penis, scrotum or testes.

kidney against the ribcage, whereas a rapid deceleration can result in renal vascular or pelviureteric injury. However, in the urban setting, penetrating trauma may account for over 20% of injuries.

History

The mechanism of trauma helps to determine which patients require urgent radiographic imaging. The degree and cause of any pre-existing renal disease may affect the chosen management (e.g. chronic renal dysfunction, renal calculi) and can predispose to injury (e.g. pelviureteric junction [PUJ] obstruction, renal cysts).

Examination

The initial examination should be focused

on cardiorespiratory findings as per the Advanced Trauma Life Support® (ATLS®) guidelines. Bruising, penetrating trauma wounds, loin or abdominal masses or fractured ribs may be detectable and may signify an underlying renal injury. Haematuria is not sensitive or specific (13% of patients with penetrating renal injury have no haematuria; conversely, 63% of patients with multi-system trauma may have haematuria, of which only about 12.5% have a confirmed renal injury). All patients suffering high-impact trauma should undergo examination of the perineum and genitalia, and have a digital rectal examination with the findings recorded in the medical records.

Investigation

Indications for computed tomography (CT) with contrast to characterise renal injury are shown in Box 5.2. Injuries can then be classified according to the American Association for the Surgery of Trauma (**Figure 5.1**). Whilst this is a useful anatomical grading system, it does not include a description of whether or not there is any active bleeding or pseudoaneurysm present. These are important features that often dictate management.

Trauma CT imaging protocols vary between hospitals. Unenhanced images will show haematomas or fluid collections although many institutions reduce the overall radiation dose by omitting this phase. An arterial phase is important to evaluate arterial bleeds and pseudoaneurysm formation. A venous phase will give information on renal parenchymal enhancement and show contusions as well as slow venous bleeds. Where a collecting system, ureteric or bladder injury is

Box 5.2 Indications for contrast-enhanced CT in the diagnosis of renal trauma.

- Blunt trauma and visible haematuria.
- Blunt trauma, non-visible haematuria and shock (systolic blood pressure <90mmHg).
- Major deceleration injury.
- Visible or non-visible haematuria after penetrating trauma.
- Paediatric trauma in a patient with visible or non-visible haematuria.
- Associated injuries suggesting underlying renal injury.

suspected, a delayed phase, usually at 10 minutes can be added. At this time the intravenous (IV) contrast medium is excreted into the collecting system. Images from a traumatic renal injury with non-contrast, arterial and venous phases are shown in **Figure 5.2**. Due to hypotension, hypovolaemia or renal injury, excretion may be impaired, so further delayed images may be necessary. Contrast medium can also be injected directly into the urinary bladder via a urethral catheter to perform a direct CT cystogram.

The intra-operative diagnosis of ureteric injuries requires a high index of suspicion. IV indigo carmine or methylene blue, or retrograde studies with fluoroscopy can be used to confirm the diagnosis. Post-operatively, any drain fluid with creatinine levels higher than serum might indicate urinary leakage. Ureteric injuries may

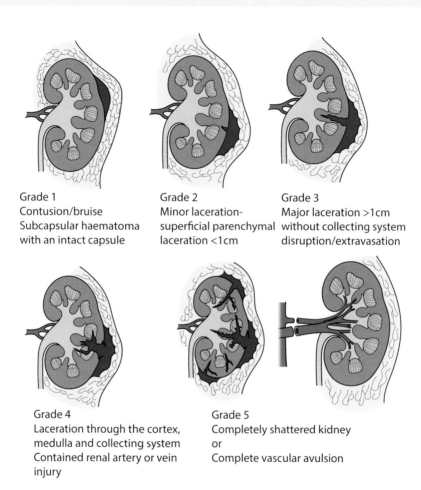

Grade 1
Contusion/bruise
Subcapsular haematoma
with an intact capsule

Grade 2
Minor laceration-
superficial parenchymal
laceration <1cm

Grade 3
Major laceration >1cm
without collecting system
disruption/extravasation

Grade 4
Laceration through the cortex,
medulla and collecting system
Contained renal artery or vein
injury

Grade 5
Completely shattered kidney
or
Complete vascular avulsion

Figure 5.1 Grades of renal trauma (American Association for the Surgery of Trauma). Advance one grade for bilateral injuries up to grade 3.

be classified according to the American Association for the Surgery of Trauma, as shown in *Box 5.3*.

Management

Renal trauma

The immediate management of renal trauma follows the ATLS® guidelines.

Subsequently, the over-riding aims are to minimise morbidity and preserve renal function. Conservative management is now commonplace, especially for patients with stable grade 1–4 blunt renal trauma and stable grade 1–3 penetrating renal trauma. Conservative management entails bed rest, prophylactic antibiotics and monitoring of vital signs. Repeat imaging

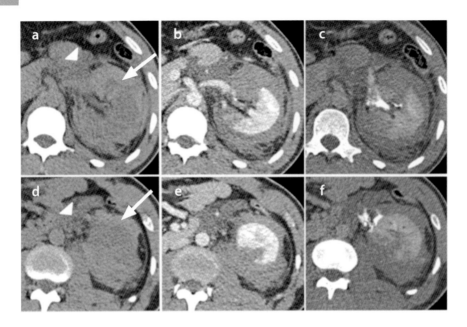

Figure 5.2 Axial computed tomography images with a non-contrast, arterial phase and delayed phase, respectively, at the level of the left renal pelvis (**a–c**) and level of the lower pole (**d–f**), showing a high-density perinephric haematoma (thin arrow) and low-density fluid collection (arrow head). The low-density fluid is shown to be a urinoma on the delayed phase images (**c** and **f**).

should be considered after 2–4 days. Eighty to ninety percent of urinary extravasation heals spontaneously but sometimes requires placement of a ureteric stent and percutaneous drain. Such management of a collecting system injury is shown in **Figure 5.3**. Percutaneous nephrostomy and/or antegrade ureteric stent insertion is possible; however, the collecting system is usually not dilated and puncture of the collecting system can be very challenging in an injured kidney.

Indications for operative or radiological management include life-threatening hae-modynamic instability, active bleeding, pseudoaneurysm, grade 5 renal injuries particularly with active bleeding, surgical exploration for associated injuries or an expanding peri-renal haematoma identi-fied during laparotomy.

Endovascular intervention is a minimally invasive option for treating arterial injury following trauma. More often than not, embolisation can be very specific in order to stop bleeding yet preserve renal function, as shown in **Figure 5.4**. It is also possible in severe injuries to perform complete embolisation of the main renal artery.

The main approach to operative management is via a midline, trans-peritoneal approach with control of the renal pedicle prior to opening the retroperitoneum. Any devitalised tissue

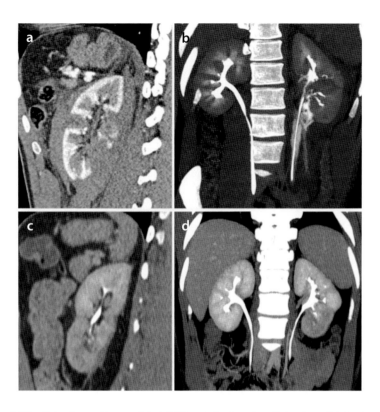

Figure 5.3 Sagittal and coronal images of the left kidney at the time of renal injury (**a** and **b**) showing a grade 4 injury with collecting system rupture, and at 3 months (**c** and **d**) showing renal preservation with lower pole scarring following conservative management and ureteric stenting.

should be debrided and if feasible, a partial nephrectomy may be performed, although the priority is to save life over preventing renal loss. If there has been damage to the collecting system this should be repaired.

Longer-term follow-up of renal trauma includes a renogram (DMSA) and ultrasound scan, usually after 3 months, to document functional and structural outcome. Serum creatinine should be checked and blood pressure monitored for the detection of possible renovascular hypertension.

Ureteric trauma

Management of ureteric trauma depends upon the timing of diagnosis, the anatomical location and the grade of the injury (*Box 5.3*). The first principle is to establish low-pressure urinary drainage either by ureteric stenting or nephrostomy placement. The optimal timing of any definitive surgical repair is not clear but should generally be considered either early (within 1 week of injury), or delayed (after 3 months) once inflammation and oedema have resolved. Surgical approaches commonly include primary repair (ureteroureterostomy),

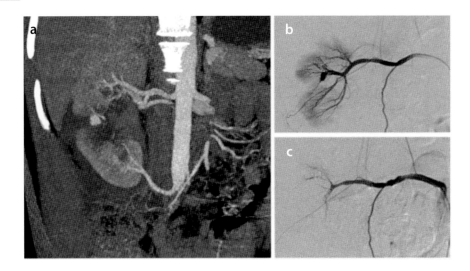

Figure 5.4 Coronal computed tomography (**a**) showing a grade 4 renal injury with a pseudoaneurysm and haematoma. Note multiple renal arteries. Digital subtraction angiograms (**b**) showing the interpolar artery supplying the pseudoaneurysm and (**c**) following super-selective embolisation.

reimplantation to either the renal pelvis (rarely a lower pole calyx) or to the bladder (psoas hitch or Boari flap). Other surgical approaches include reimplantation of the affected ureter into the contralateral ureter (transureteroureterostomy), auto-transplantation of the entire kidney and ureter, an ileal interposition graft that can replace part of, or the whole ureter, or performing a nephrectomy.

A successful ureteric repair relies upon a tension-free anastomosis of viable tissue. Spatulation of the distal and proximal ureteric ends is recommended to reduce the chance of stricture formation. An internal stent and external non-suction drain are placed, and if possible the repair covered with peritoneum or omentum.

Box 5.3 The American Association for the Surgery of Trauma: grades of ureteric trauma.

- Grade I – haematoma.
- Grade 2 – laceration <50% circumference.
- Grade 3 – laceration >50% circumference.
- Grade 4 – complete transection with <2cm of devascularisation.
- Grade 5 – complete transection with >2cm of devascularisation.
- Advance one grade for bilateral injuries up to grade 3.

LOWER URINARY TRACT TRAUMA

Lower urinary tract trauma encompasses trauma to the bladder or urethra.

Causes

Causes of lower urinary tract trauma are summarised in *Box 5.4*.

Bladder injuries can be classified as blunt, penetrating or iatrogenic. Eighty percent of traumatic ruptures are associated with pelvic fractures. Rupture may occur into the peritoneum (40% of cases) or the retroperitoneum (60%). Peritoneal rupture usually occurs after a sudden increase in bladder pressure where the bladder ruptures through the weakest part, the dome. Extraperitoneal bladder rupture is also strongly associated with pelvic fractures. Iatrogenic bladder injury can be a complication of hysterectomy, Caesarean section and transurethral resection of a bladder tumour.

Urethral trauma is more common in men and associated either with blunt or iatrogenic injury in most cases. The anterior urethra (distal to the urogenital diaphragm) is exposed and therefore at risk from blunt trauma, especially in 'fall-astride' injuries. More commonly, injuries can occur from urethral instrumentation and catheterisation. Penile fracture is a rarer cause of anterior urethral trauma (page 79). The posterior urethra is almost exclusively injured with concomitant pelvic fractures, seen in up to 19% of male pelvic fractures.

Box **5.4** Causes of lower urinary tract injuries.

Bladder

- Blunt: associated with pelvic fractures.

- Penetrating: rare.

- Iatrogenic: cystoscopic procedures, particularly transurethral resection of bladder tumours, pelvic cancer surgery and gynaecological surgery.

Urethra

- Anterior: associated with blunt trauma and instrumentation.

- Posterior: associated with pelvic fractures.

Presentation

Bladder injuries
Visible haematuria is seen in up to 95% of cases. Urinary retention and suprapubic pain are also common symptoms. Intraperitoneal rupture may also be associated with the development of an ileus, abdominal distension, urinary ascites or an unexplained elevation in serum creatinine.

Urethral injuries
Blood at the urethral meatus is the hallmark of urethral injury. It is present in 37–93% of posterior and at least 75% of anterior urethral injuries. Urinary retention, penile and/or perineal haematoma and a high-riding prostate on rectal examination may support the diagnosis. If a urethral injury is suspected, one cautious attempt at catheterisation by an experienced doctor

is permissible. However, if the catheter does not pass, a urethrogram should be performed and a suprapubic catheter placed if a urethral injury is confirmed.

Patterns of haematoma associated with anterior urethral injury
Anterior urethral injuries from perineal trauma often result in haematoma and a pattern of bruising that is either confined to the penis or may extend in a 'butterfly' pattern to involve the perineum and buttocks. The pattern and extent of the haematoma is determined by the attachments of the fascial layers of the penis, perineum and abdominal wall. Injury to the anterior urethra that does not lead to disruption of the integrity of the deeper Buck's fascia results in a haematoma that is limited to the penis. Where Buck's fascia is disrupted, the haematoma extends freely within the perineum in a 'butterfly' pattern and is limited only by the attachment of the more superficial Colles' fascia to the ischial tuberosities (**Figure 5.5**). It may also extend onto the anterior abdominal wall and chest corresponding to the superior limits of Scarpa's fascia (**Figure 5.6**).

Investigation
To diagnose bladder injuries a cystogram is the investigation of choice. This can be indirect during a delayed phase of the trauma CT, direct by filling the bladder and CT imaging (as shown in **Figure 5.7**) or direct, by filling the bladder under fluoroscopic control. Filling of the retrovesical space, paracolic gutters and outlining of intra-abdominal viscera are indicative of intraperitoneal rupture. Extraperitoneal rupture is associated with characteristic 'flame-shaped' areas of extravasation confined to the peri-

Figure 5.5 Scrotal and perineal bruising after a 'straddle' injury. Image used with permission of Elsevier Ltd. Bullock N, Doble A, Turner WH, Cuckow P. *Urology: An Illustrated Colour Text*. Elsevier, Churchill Livingstone, 2007; p49, Fig. 3.

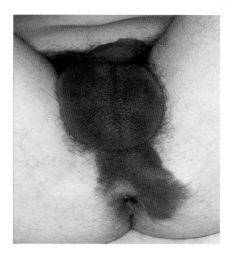

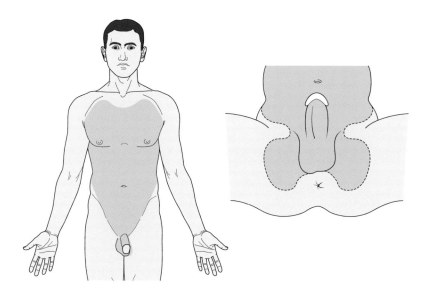

Figure 5.6 Diagram demonstrating the potential haematoma pattern caused by a urethral injury with an accompanying tear to Buck's fascia. This classically leads to a butterfly haematoma across the perineum, and extension of blood through the penis, scrotum and lower abdominal wall. If Buck's fascia remains intact, haematoma is limited to the penis.

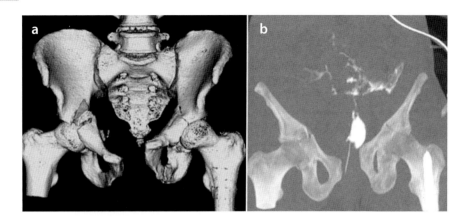

Figure 5.7 3D shaded surface computed tomography (CT) reconstruction (**a**) showing an 'open book'-type pelvic fracture. Corresponding coronal direct CT cystogram (**b**) showing a high-riding displaced bladder with an intraperitoneal rupture and leak of contrast medium.

vesical tissue and occasionally a so-called 'teardrop deformity' caused by a large pelvic haematoma.

Urethral injuries are best diagnosed with retrograde urethrography, performed using a 14 Fr Foley catheter inserted into the distal urethra, with the balloon inflated in the fossa navicularis using 1–2ml of water. Undiluted contrast (20–30ml) is injected and radiographs taken in a 30° oblique position. Retrograde urethrography highlighting a posterior urethral injury following pelvic trauma is shown in **Figure 5.8**. This test is inappropriate in unstable patients who would benefit primarily from image-guided suprapubic catheter insertion.

Management

If a suprapubic catheter is required, this should be placed using a Seldinger technique under ultrasound guidance by a doctor experienced in the technique. The skin insertion point must be in the midline and should be 2–3 fingerbreadths above the symphysis pubis. A 16 Fr silicone catheter should be used. Bladder injuries associated with a normal cystogram are usually attributable to a peri-vesical haematoma and conservative management with catheter drainage alone is appropriate. Similarly, the majority of patients with an extraperitoneal rupture can be managed with a urethral catheter. The exceptions to this include patients with bladder neck or associated vaginal or rectal injuries and those undergoing operative repair of a pelvic fracture, particularly where a bony spicule penetrates the bladder. External penetrating injuries and blunt intraperitoneal bladder ruptures require formal surgical exploration and open repair. Absorbable sutures are mandatory in order to prevent subsequent bladder stones and it is generally advisable to leave both a suprapubic and urethral catheter. Most surgeons advocate performing a follow-up cystogram 10–14 days later prior to catheter removal.

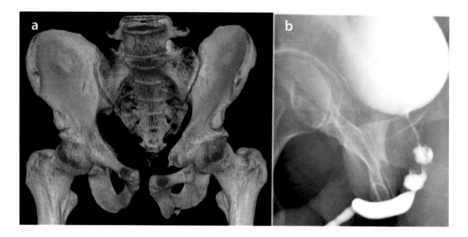

Figure 5.8 3D shaded surface computed tomography reconstruction (**a**) showing a pelvic fracture. A retrograde urethrogram (**b**) showing a posterior urethral injury with a leak of contrast medium from the membranous urethra.

Indications for primary (within 48 hours) urethral repair are: associated anorectal injury, perineal degloving, bladder neck injury, massive bladder displacement and penetrating trauma to the anterior urethra. This complex surgery should be undertaken in a specialist centre by a surgeon specialising in reconstructive urology. Primary realignment of the urethra during fracture surgery is no longer recommended, as in the hands of an inexperienced surgeon the risk of additional damage probably outweighs the benefits. Accurate reduction of the bony pelvic ring indirectly realigns the urethra and facilitates delayed repair. Delayed repair should be carried out 3 months post-injury by a reconstructive urological surgeon.

Key Points

- 80% of traumatic bladder ruptures are associated with pelvic fractures.
- Visible haematuria is present in up to 95% of cases of bladder trauma.
- A cystogram is the investigation of choice to investigate bladder rupture.
- In trauma cases, check for blood at the urethral meatus; this is a sign of urethral injury.
- Blood at the meatus is seen in 37–93% of posterior and at least 75% of anterior urethral injuries.
- A retrograde urethrogram is the investigation of choice for urethral injury.

GENITOSCROTAL TRAUMA

Genital trauma refers to injury to the male or female sex organs, especially those outside the body.

Despite the seemingly vulnerable position of the male genitalia within the scrotum, traumatic injury is relatively rare. Genital injury may be very painful and associated with significant bleeding. Genital injury may have an effect on fertility and therefore requires urgent attention.

Trauma to female genitalia is best managed by gynaecological specialists. The following relates to male genitalia only.

Testicular trauma

Testicular trauma may be categorised as blunt, penetrating or degloving. Blunt trauma to the testis can occur from a kick to the groin or from being struck by a hard object such as a cricket ball. Blunt injuries are more common (approximately 85%) than penetrating injuries and are frequently minor, often permitting a conservative management approach. Penetrating injury from sharp objects or gun shot typically require surgical exploration and treatment, and in these instances bilateral injury is much more common. Degloving refers to shearing of the scrotal skin and dartos muscle leaving the testes exposed. Dislocation of the testis from its orthotopic (normal) position within the scrotum typically occurs in motorcycle accidents where impact with the fuel tank forces the testis into the inguinal canal (**Figure 5.9**). Treatment is by manual closed reduction and surgical fixation if necessary.

Presentation

- Patients experiencing testicular trauma are usually able to give a clear history of the mechanism of injury and report severe pain and swelling of the genitalia. They may have associated nausea and vomiting.
- Examination often reveals a swollen and tender testis. It is important to confirm the presence of a normal contralateral testis, although bilateral injury is quite rare. The perineum should be examined to exclude associated injuries.
- A detailed history and examination should allow exclusion of differential diagnoses such as epididymo-orchitis and testicular torsion.
- Penetrating injuries require particular attention to entry and exit wounds and evaluation for associated femoral vascular injury.

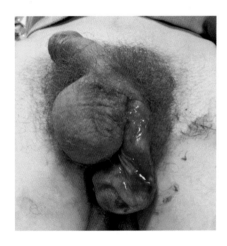

Figure 5.9 Clinical image of a young motorcyclist involved in a road traffic collision. The left testicle has extruded through the ruptured scrotum but remains viable. An unusual injury.

Investigation

Urinalysis may help to exclude an infective cause. Ultrasonography with Doppler studies is extremely valuable in the evaluation of testicular injuries. Ultrasound may show blood within the parietal tunica vaginalis (haematocoele). Disruption of the tunica albuginea (outer casing) of the testis, often with associated haematocoele, is pathognomonic for testicular rupture (**Figure 5.10**). Doppler studies also allow assessment of the vascular integrity of the testis and absence of flow may indicate torsion or devascularisation of the spermatic cord. Where there remains uncertainty regarding the diagnosis, surgical exploration may be the best diagnostic investigation.

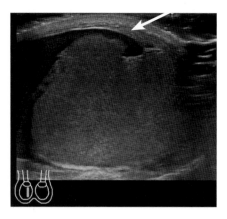

Figure 5.10 Testicular rupture following trauma sustained while playing football. Disruption of the tunica albuginea with extrusion of seminiferous tubules can be seen with a small associated haematocoele.

Management

A conservative management approach, with scrotal support and non-steroidal anti-inflammatories may be adopted where there is no scrotal violation and the testis is explicitly normal. Haematocoeles no larger than three times the size of the contralateral testis should be managed non-operatively. Larger haematocoeles, even where the tunica albuginea is intact, should be explored surgically as expedient operative intervention may lead to lower rates of orchidectomy. Small intratesticular haematomas can be managed conservatively (**Figure 5.11**). However, it should be noted that where the tunica albuginea is intact, even small

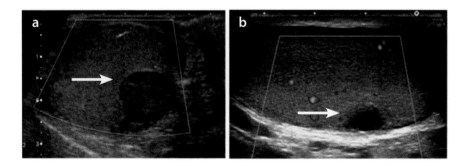

Figure 5.11 (**a**) Ultrasound image showing a 33mm intratesticular haematoma following trauma sustained during martial arts combat. (**b**) A repeat scan 4 weeks later following conservative management shows the haematoma has reduced in size to only 7mm.

intratesticular haematomas may result in significantly raised pressures that can lead to necrosis and later atrophy. Indications for surgical exploration are given in *Box 5.5*.

Disruption of the tunica albuginea (testicular rupture) requires urgent surgical exploration and repair. Delayed treatment or conservative management may lead to loss of endocrine and/or spermatogenic function and is more likely to result in testicular atrophy and later orchidectomy.

Box 5.5 Indications for surgical exploration in testicular trauma.

- Disruption of tunica albuginea.
- Ambiguity regarding diagnosis.
- Large or expanding haematocoele.
- Penetrating trauma.
- Degloving injury.
- Testicular dislocation.

Surgical approach

The tunica vaginalis is opened and the haematoma evacuated (**Figure 5.12**). Devitalised extruded seminiferous tubules are debrided and the tunica albuginea closed with absorbable sutures. Wound irrigation followed by insertion of a dependent drain and broad-spectrum antibiotics are required. Orchidectomy is rarely needed except in cases of a shattered testis or testicular infarction. In cases of degloving, primary closure of the scrotum is favoured following copious irrigation. Where scrotal tissue loss is extensive (>80%), closure may not be possible, and instead the testes may be placed within medial thigh pouches.

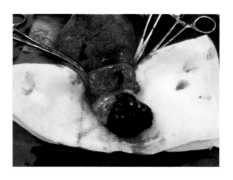

Figure 5.12 Intra-operative appearances of testicular rupture: the tunica vaginalis has been everted to show the ruptured tunica albuginea of the testis with haematoma and extruded seminiferous tubules.

Zipper injury

Penile zipper injuries generally refer to entrapment of the prepuce of uncircumcised males in the fly zipper of their trousers. There is rarely any significant delay in presentation because of the pain and entrapment. Rarely, delayed presentation can result in infection and potentially development of Fournier's gangrene. Prophylactic antibiotics should be administered. Children are often in pain and may be agitated and it is therefore important to ensure adequate pain relief.

In adults it may be possible to attempt disengagement of the foreskin from the zipper using local anaesthesia, but in children sedation or general anaesthesia is usually required. Knowledge of the anatomy and mechanics of the zipper is essential to ensure safe and effective treatment. The zipper is a slide fastener with anterior and posterior face plates connected by a median bar that moves along metal or plastic teeth of the zipper (**Figure 5.13**).

Where the foreskin is caught between the zip teeth, away from the zipper itself, the foreskin may be released by cutting through the zip below and disengaging the teeth. However, where the penis is entrapped within the zipper mechanism itself, a number of different techniques may be considered. It is generally inadvisable to simply try to unzip the zipper as this is likely to cause more tissue damage. Although mineral oil to provide lubrication has been used to successfully extricate the entrapped foreskin, it is generally advisable to release the zipper mechanism itself. This can be achieved using a pair of orthopaedic bone cutters to divide the median bar that connects the two face plates (**Figure 5.13**). This allows the two face plates to separate and the zipper teeth to disengage with the release of the ensnared tissue. Alternatively, a screwdriver or similar instrument can be inserted between the face plates, and a twisting motion used to prise them apart with the concomitant release of the zipper teeth and foreskin. An emergency circumcision should only be considered in exceptional circumstances.

Penile trauma

Penile fracture is covered in Chapter 4 (page 79). Other types of penile trauma include amputation, penetrating injury and soft tissue injury.

Penile amputation

A significant proportion of penile amputations occur as a result of psychotic mental illness, most commonly schizophrenia. Another common cause is disorders of gender identity leading individuals to attempt gender conversion.

Management

Acute psychosis must be urgently treated through the involvement of a psychiatrist. Where the amputated penis has been salvaged, it should be cleaned and wrapped in saline-soaked gauze before being placed on ice to reduce ischaemic injury. It should not, however, be immersed in the ice mix. Reattachment should be undertaken as soon as possible at a centre with specialist reconstructive expertise.

Any devitalised tissue should be debrided and adequate exposure obtained. The urethra is first anastomosed over a Foley catheter using a 4/0 or 5/0 absorbable suture. Some surgeons advocate microvascular repair of the deep cavernosal arteries while others do not routinely undertake this step. The tunica albuginea of the corpora cavernosa are then repaired using a 2/0 absorbable suture. Microsurgical repair of the dorsal neurovascular bundles

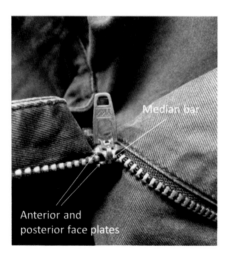

Figure 5.13 Fly zipper showing the anterior and posterior face plates connected by a median bar that moves along the metal teeth of the zipper.

is undertaken before closing the dartos fascia and lastly the skin.

The patient should be given IV antibiotics initially before completing an oral course. The role of anticoagulation is somewhat controversial. Some believe that it helps to maintain patency of the anastomosed penile vasculature, while others consider the risk of haematoma outweighs any potential benefit.

The long-term outcomes are relatively good with more than 80% retaining some erectile function and sensation. Urethral strictures occur in approximately 20% of patients.

Penetrating injury

Penetrating penile injuries usually occur during wartime conflicts and are the result of shrapnel, bullet or stab wounds. They may involve the urethra and/or corpora cavernosa. Blood at the urethral meatus may signify a urethral injury and prompt investigation by means of a urethrogram.

Surgical repair should be undertaken as soon as possible with debridement of devitalised tissue and reconstruction. Exposure may be achieved in the same way as for the treatment of penile fracture, typically with a circumferential degloving incision.

Soft tissue injury

Soft tissue penile injuries may be the result of animal or human bites, burns, mechanical trauma or that related to tissue destruction from infection (Fournier's gangrene; see Chapter 4). Expeditious surgical repair should be attempted. Necrotic tissue should be debrided and the wound irrigated with povidone iodine. With the exception of human bites that are at very high risk of infection, the wound should be closed, with skin grafts used to cover larger defects. Broad-spectrum antibiotics should be administered as prophylaxis for human and animal bites and where there is evidence of infection in other cases.

Key Points

- Ultrasound has an important role in the diagnosis and management of testicular trauma but there should be a low threshold for surgical exploration where there remains diagnostic uncertainty.
- Knowledge of the mechanics of the fly zipper is essential to ensure safe and effective treatment of penile skin entrapment.
- Consider early involvement of a specialist andrology centre with complex penile injuries.

Chapter 6
Special Circumstances

Andrew Robb[1] / Holly Weaver and Nikesh Thiruchelvam[2, 3, 4, 5, 6] / Suzanne Biers[3]

PAEDIATRIC UROLOGICAL EMERGENCIES[1]

Urological emergencies in childhood are common. In this chapter we discuss a number of the more common emergencies encountered.

Acute scrotum in childhood

Defined as an acute onset of painful swelling of the scrotum or its contents. It is the commonest urological emergency encountered in children. The causes of an acute scrotum are listed in *Box 6.1*. Irreversible damage to the testicle can be observed after 4 hours of ischaemia; therefore, testicular torsion and incarcerated inguinal hernia must be rapidly identified and treated.

Testicular torsion

Although testicular torsion has a bimodal incidence it may present at any time in childhood. The peak incidence occurs during:

- The perinatal period (neonatal torsion).
- Early puberty.

Box 6.1 Differential diagnosis of the acute scrotum in children.

- Testicular torsion.
- Torted appendages.
- Infection.
- Idiopathic scrotal oedema.
- Trauma.
- Incarcerated inguinal hernia.
- Henoch-Schönlein purpura.
- Haematological malignancy.

Testicular torsion often presents in a manner similar to that in adults (see page 69). In children it can also have an atypical presentation, with the child complaining of abdominal or loin pain. Abdominal examination in all paediatric patients should include examination of the external genitalia for this reason.

The use of ultrasonography is controversial. It may be helpful in establishing or excluding a diagnosis in difficult cases. However, it may cause undue delay in getting a patient to theatre for treatment of the torsion.

Treatment is emergency scrotal exploration (see also page 71). A midline (median raphe) incision or transverse scrotal incision may be employed. The tunica vaginalis (sac of tissue around the testis) is opened to expose the affected testicle. If a testicular torsion is identified, it should be untwisted and left for several minutes in a warm saline-soaked gauze and re-assessed for viability. For proven cases of torsion, both testes should be fixed (bilateral orchidopexy) to prevent further episodes of torsion (and ischaemia) on either the affected side or the contralateral 'normal' side. The contralateral testis may be particularly susceptible to torsion due to cord insertion in the interpolar region of the testis leading to a 'bell-clapper' configuration. If the testis is no longer viable due to prolonged torsion, removal of the testis is required (orchidectomy), along with fixation of the other testis. Manual attempts to try to untwist the testis directly through the scrotal skin (scrotal detorsion) has no role in the management of testicular torsion.

Neonatal testicular torsion

In this clinical scenario, the torsion event happens before or around the time of birth. The presentation will depend on the time before birth that the torsion occurred:

- Prolonged period before birth: the infant may be born with an absent testis, and should be managed as a patient with an impalpable testis.
- Weeks before birth: the infant may present with a regular, firm, painless mass that is smaller than the normal contralateral testis. The mass is attached to the scrotal wall and there is no evidence of acute inflammation.
- Days or hours before birth: a painful enlarged testis with overlying inflammatory changes in the scrotal wall is seen.
- If the torsion occurs after birth, the scrotum will appear normal on initial inspection, but acute inflammatory signs will develop later.

Management is controversial. Some surgeons explore all neonates with evidence of torsion; others manage all patients conservatively except for neonates who present with acute symptoms after birth. The option of a contralateral orchidopexy should be discussed with the parents.

Torted testicular appendage

This is the commonest reason for scrotal exploration in childhood, particularly in pre-pubertal boys. The testicular appendage (also known as the hydatid of Morgagni) is a small tissue remnant found at the superior pole of the testis in most males. It is often pedunculated and therefore prone to torsion. If it twists it causes oedema and venous congestion, leading to ischaemia and infarction of the appendage, which manifests as pain.

On clinical examination, a blue spot (Figure 4.2, page 72) may be visible through the scrotum (in around a third of cases), and the clinician may be able to elicit point tenderness over the upper pole of the testis.

It is a self-limiting condition with resolution of symptoms typically after 3–5 days. It can therefore be managed conservatively with rest and analgesia. Alternatively, scrotal exploration can be performed with immediate resolution of symptoms.

After taking a history and examination, if there is any concern or residual doubt that the patient may have a testicular torsion, the patient should have an emergency scrotal exploration.

Infection

Epididymitis or orchitis can occur in both pre- and post-pubertal boys. Presentation is similar to that seen in adults. A urine dipstick should be performed and urine culture sent. Doppler ultrasound may reveal an enlarged testis with increased blood flow to the epididymis or testicle compared to the contralateral side.

If any doubt regarding the diagnosis exists, scrotal exploration is mandatory. Following diagnosis, treatment is with appropriate antibiotics.

Trauma

Scrotal trauma is relatively common in boys and may be caused by a direct blow or a straddle injury. Trauma may precipitate testicular torsion, so it is important not to overlook this diagnosis.

Assessment by ultrasonography may demonstrate the presence of haematoma or testicular rupture. A haematoma can be managed conservatively, whilst a ruptured testicle should be repaired.

Idiopathic scrotal oedema

Idiopathic scrotal oedema is a condition seen in pre-pubertal males. The peak incidence occurs between 5 and 6 years of age. As the name suggests, the cause is unknown. It is characterised by swelling of the scrotum and redness (**Figure 6.1**). This may occur unilaterally or bilaterally, and it may extend upward into the inguinal region or to the perineum (often seen as a red inverted triangle in the perineum).

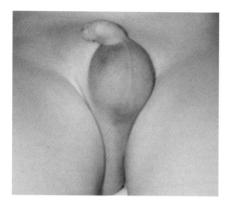

Figure 6.1 Idiopathic scrotal oedema.

Importantly the testes themselves are not tender on examination.

The condition resolves spontaneously, often within 24–48 hours. No specific treatment is required. Antihistamines or antibiotics are sometimes prescribed, but there is no good evidence to support their use.

Henoch–Schönlein purpura (HSP)

This is an acute immunoglobulin-A (IgA)-mediated vasculitis that presents with a typical rash on the legs. Involvement of the scrotum and testis in HSP is a well-documented complication. It gives rise to acute tenderness, swelling and scrotal discolouration. Scrotal exploration is not required.

Penile and foreskin problems in children

Post-circumcision complications

Complications following circumcision are common, and include:

- Bleeding. Initially, circumferential pressure around the penis should be applied. If this fails then exploration and revision of circumcision under general anaesthesia (GA) is needed. The patient should also be investigated for a bleeding diathesis.

- Retained PlastiBell® (plastic device used for neonatal circumcision). This may require a short GA to remove the retained device.
- Glans trauma. This should be referred to a paediatric urologist for further management, as it may require specialist repair under GA.
- Excess skin removed. This should be referred to a paediatric urologist for further management, as it may need formal reconstruction.

Paraphimosis

Paraphimosis is caused by the foreskin being retracted and cannot then return to its normal position (**Figure 6.2**). It can result in injury or necrosis of the foreskin (and the glans). It may present with pain or acute urinary obstruction. The diagnosis should be obvious on examination.

The foreskin should be reduced as soon as possible. Manual reduction is achieved by reducing the oedema from the foreskin.

It is then replaced by using the thumbs to push down on the glans while the other fingers pull the foreskin forwards into its anatomical position. Adequate analgesia should be given prior to reduction.

It may be necessary to perform this under GA in children. If manual reduction under GA fails, then a dorsal slit can be employed. Although it is an option in an adult patient, circumcision should not be performed in the acute setting if possible due to the high complication rate.

Voiding problems in children

Urinary retention

Urinary retention in childhood is uncommon. There are a large number of causes (*Box 6.2*). Urinary retention should be looked at as a symptom that requires identification of the underlying cause. Dependent on the aetiology, urinary retention may be painful or painless.

Box 6.2 Causes of urinary retention in childhood.

- Post-operative.
- Urinary tract infection (UTI).
- Balanitis xerotica obliterans.
- Constipation.
- Drugs.
- Bladder outlet obstruction.
- Neurological.
- Voiding dysfunction.
- Neoplasm.
- Idiopathic.

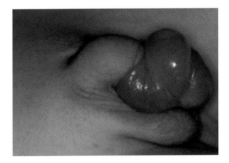

Figure 6.2 Paraphimosis.

Assessment includes a full history, full physical examination including neurological examination, assessment of the spine and sacrum, and examination of external genitalia. A rectal examination should also be considered where clinically appropriate, preferably after paediatric urology review, and deferred where possible to be performed under GA if the child is also having a cystoscopy or other intervention.

Treatment involves ensuring adequate drainage of the bladder and treating the underlying cause of the retention. Options for achieving drainage of the bladder include:

- Spontaneous voiding.
- Getting the child to relax (playing in the bath is a good strategy).
- Benzodiazepines may help.
- Urethral catheterisation.
- Suprapubic catheterisation.

Balanitis xerotica obliterans (BXO) is a benign, scarring condition that can affect the foreskin, glans of the penis and urethra (**Figure 6.3**). Most commonly it causes a pathological phimosis (tightening) of the foreskin, but it can also cause narrowing of the external urethral meatus and urethral strictures. If BXO is identified as the cause of urinary retention, then an emergency circumcision is required (with further treatment of any associated meatal stenosis or urethral stricture disease if identified).

In all cases of urinary retention the case should be discussed with a specialist paediatric urologist.

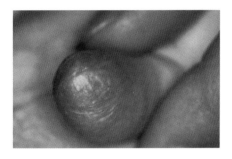

Figure 6.3 Balanitis xerotica obliterans as a cause of acute urinary retention.

Key Points

- Testicular torsion in children can have an atypical presentation, necessitating examination of genitalia in all paediatric patients with abdominal pain.
- Procedures in children may require general anaesthesia.
- Urinary retention in childhood requires specialist paediatric urology input.

UROLOGICAL EMERGENCIES IN PREGNANCY[2]

Although pregnant women may seek medical attention for a range of pregnancy-related problems, they can still be affected by the full range of urological diseases that may affect them in their non-pregnant state. Several important factors must be taken into consideration when approaching urological disease in the pregnant woman. Firstly, awareness of the stage of pregnancy and ongoing dialogue with the obstetric team are crucial. This is particularly pertinent when deciding management options, to ensure medical treatments and surgical interventions are safe in pregnancy. This also means the range of investigations and management options are limited compared to the non-pregnant patient, as the well-being of the fetus is paramount. Secondly, interpretation of investigation results must be done with the knowledge of the physiological and anatomical changes affecting the urinary system in pregnancy, to best inform management decisions (*Box 6.3*). Of particular note, there is progressive dilatation of the renal collecting system known as a physiological hydronephrosis. This is classically more pronounced on the right side than the left (**Figure 6.4**), which can make the diagnosis of new pathological hydronephrosis difficult to identify.

Pyelonephritis in pregnancy

Pyelonephritis occurs in up to 1 in every 50 pregnancies with recognised obstetric complications including pre-term labour, pre-eclampsia and low birth weight. The prevalence of asymptomatic bacteriuria is comparable with the non-pregnant population, but more pregnant women go on to develop symptoms and upper UTI (pyelonephitis), due to a dilated collecting system and urinary stasis promoting bacterial growth. Women should be screened for asymptomatic bacteriuria frequently in pregnancy, and treated where positive. They should also be treated quickly and effectively if pyelonephritis is suspected. The physiological changes of pregnancy can mask signs of sepsis, and as pregnant women can deteriorate very rapidly, any delay in treatment may have harmful consequences.

Box 6.3 Changes to the urinary system in pregnancy.

- Kidneys enlarge due to increased intravascular volume.

- Dilatation of the renal pelvis (physiological hydronephrosis) and hydroureter due to hormonal muscle relaxants and pressure from the gravid uterus.

- Glomerular filtration rate increases by up to half, so urea and creatinine levels will be lower than the reference range for the non-pregnant woman.

- Bladder tone decreases and capacity increases.

- With uterine growth, urinary frequency, urgency, nocturia and incontinence become more common.

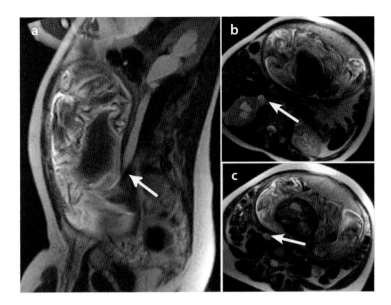

Figure 6.4 Physiological hydronephrosis of pregnancy. T2-weighted magnetic resonance imaging with sagittal view (**a**) showing a right-sided hydronephrosis and hydroureter due to compression of the ureter at the pelvic brim as a result of the gravid uterus (arrow). Axial images also show the right hydronephrosis and dilated upper ureter (**b**) and dilated right ureter below the kidney (**c**).

History
- Stage of pregnancy with an up-to-date obstetric history.
- Onset and nature of symptoms: loin tenderness, dysuria, fever.
- Screen for obstetric complications: discharge or bleeding per vagina.

Examination
Depending on the stage of pregnancy, the gravid uterus may make examination more difficult, but a thorough examination is still important, particularly to elicit any flank tenderness.

Ensure appropriate obstetric support for the antenatal mother and fetal checks.

Investigation
- Bloods: as for non-pregnant cases of suspected pyelonephritis, taking into account the physiological change in blood result parameters (creatinine and urea lower due to a higher GFR).
- Urine dip and culture.
- Blood cultures.
- Imaging: an ultrasound scan of the kidneys, ureters, bladder (USS KUB) can be performed, but interpretation needs to account for the physiological hydronephrosis of pregnancy. Computed tomography (CT) is avoided due to the radiation exposure risk to the fetus.

Management in moderate to severe pyelonephritis

- Aggressive intravenous (IV) fluid resuscitation.
- Timely and safe IV antibiotics after cultures are taken. Discuss with both the obstetric team and microbiology to use an effective antibiotic that is safe for the stage of pregnancy and/or consult your national drug formulary. Empirical antibiotics are started until the urine culture results are known.
- If systemic inflammatory response syndrome (SIRS) criteria are met (see page 12), the patient will need the 'Sepsis Six Bundle' as they would in the non-pregnant state (see page 14).
- Ongoing assessment and management of both the mother and the fetal parameters are needed throughout with obstetric input.
- Once the infection is controlled (i.e. temperature and other observations have settled with IV antibiotics), the patient should complete a prolonged course of oral antibiotics (typically to complete a total of 10 days therapy), guided by the urine cultures.
- For the duration of the pregnancy, a repeat urine dipstick and/or cultures should be regularly checked at antenatal visits.

Acute kidney injury in pregnancy

Causes of acute kidney injury (AKI) in pregnancy can be classified as pre-renal, intrinsic or post-renal in origin, as for the non-pregnant population (*Box 6.4*). However, assessment and management must take into consideration causes specific to pregnancy, such as the glomerular injury of pre-eclampsia, or the hypovolaemic state induced by obstetric haemorrhage. It is also important to remember the adjusted reference ranges for laboratory values in the pregnant population, whereby what is a slightly elevated creatinine or urea for the non-pregnant state, may actually indicate a significant deterioration in renal function in pregnancy.

History

- An up-to-date obstetric history, including any history of pre-eclampsia or hypertensive disorders in previous pregnancies.
- Any new symptoms, vomiting or hyperemesis gravidarum or other causes of volume depletion.

Box 6.4 Causes of AKI specific to pregnancy.

- Pre-renal: intravascular volume depletion secondary to haemorrhage, sepsis or vomiting.
- Intrinsic: pre-eclampsia, HELLP* syndrome.
- Post-renal: any cause of urinary tract obstruction in single kidney function or affecting urinary tracts bilaterally if normal function.

*HELLP (H, haemolysis; EL, elevated liver enzymes; LP, low platelets) syndrome is a life-threatening emergency encountered in the later stages of pregnancy, and considered a variant of pre-eclampsia. Common presentations include headache, nausea and vomiting, abdominal tenderness, and it is commonly associated with hypertension and proteinuria.

- Any known chronic renal failure. Renal function tends to deteriorate in pregnancy if there is pre-existing renal damage.

Examination
- Assess for evidence of bleeding (obstetric or otherwise) as part of the initial fluid balance assessment that could cause hypovolaemia.
- Any signs of sepsis causing intravascular fluid depletion.
- Consider pre-eclampsia as a cause of renal dysfunction: should be suspected in any hypertensive state in pregnancy and diagnosis usually involves evidence of proteinuria; may also see pitting, non-dependent oedema.

Investigation
- Bloods: note the importance of adjusted normal parameters in pregnancy; the reference range for creatinine and urea is lower than in the non-pregnant state, especially in the first trimester, so be careful not to overlook clinically significant rises.
- Imaging: USS KUB can be performed, but interpretation needs to account for the physiological hydronephrosis of pregnancy.
- Urine dipstick (look for proteinuria as well as evidence of infection).

Management
With awareness of the changes in renal physiology in pregnancy and appropriate treatment of the causes of AKI (see pages 17–21), renal function usually returns to normal.

Urolithiasis in pregnancy
The formation of calculi in the urinary tract (or urolithiasis) is a common cause for hospital admissions in pregnancy, with most presenting in the second or third trimesters. Overall, the incidence of renal colic is reported to be the same in pregnant and non-pregnant women; however, there are several factors that can contribute to stone formation in pregnancy including hypercalciuria and an increased excretion of urinary citrate (which is normally protective against stone formation). Most patients will present with flank pain. Other possible differential diagnoses also need to be checked and excluded, including pyelonephritis, appendicitis and placental complications. Stones are associated with an increased risk of pre-term labour.

History
- Stage of pregnancy with an up-to-date obstetric history.
- Onset and nature of symptoms.
- Fevers or rigors.
- Evidence of UTI/infection.
- Surgical history: remember other surgical emergencies like appendicitis can present atypically in pregnancy.
- Personal or family history of ureteric calculi.

Examination
- Abdominal exam: renal angle tenderness; check whether abdominal distension is consistent with stage of pregnancy, with obstetric input to assess mother and fetal well-being.
- Close monitoring of observations for haemodynamic instability and temperature.

Investigation

- Urinalysis and culture.
- Bloods including full blood count (FBC), C-reactive protein (CRP), renal function. Note that biochemistry reference ranges can be altered in pregnancy.
- Septic screen if febrile, hypotensive or tachycardic.
- Imaging: first-line imaging is USS. It will be able to demonstrate a non-physiological hydronephrosis and can provide a safe modality to monitor the clinical situation. It can also identify the presence of ureteric jets (if there is concern regarding an obstructed renal system). USS has a poor sensitivity for ureteric stones, but it avoids the risks of teratogenicity and childhood malignancy associated with CT.
- Any other imaging needs discussion with radiology, urology, obstetrics and the patient. Options for second-line imaging may include magnetic resonance imaging without contrast. Low-dose CT has a high sensitivity and specificity for stones, but is best avoided due to radiation exposure risk, as is single-shot intravenous pyelography.

Management

- Multi-disciplinary approach: needs ongoing discussion with obstetrics in light of potential complications and the need for intervention.
- Conservative management is the preferred first-line option with a trial of spontaneous stone passage with hydration and analgesia. Spontaneous stone passage is encouraged by ureteric smooth muscle relaxation due to higher progesterone levels.

Non-steroidal anti-inflammatory drugs (NSAIDs) should be avoided in pregnancy.

- Intervention is indicated if there is evidence of:
  › Sepsis (fever, infection).
  › Renal insufficiency, bilateral obstruction, or problems in a solitary kidney.
  › Obstetric complications relating to the stone.
  › Refractory pain, nausea and vomiting and a large stone.

Temporary drainage versus definitive treatment

- Urgent temporary drainage is indicated if fever and infection are associated with a ureteric stone (indicating an infected, obstructed system). This can be achieved with ureteric stent insertion in theatre or ultrasound-guided nephrostomy insertion.
- Ureteric stent placement demands ongoing management through pregnancy due to accelerated rates of encrustation due to hypercalciuria, and thus requires replacement every 4–6 weeks. The same applies for nephrostomy insertion.
- Intervention with ureteroscopy and removal of the stone with a basket or laser fragmentation. This avoids the need for regular stent exchanges but can be challenging.

Often it is difficult to make an accurate diagnosis because of the inability to use ionising radiation. As such, it is acceptable to offer nephrostomy drainage or ureteric stenting without a definite diagnosis of a ureteric stone until pregnancy is complete.

Treatments that are contraindicated in pregnancy are extracorporeal shock wave lithotripsy (ESWL) and percutaneous nephrolithotomy (PCNL).

NEUROGENIC BLADDER[3]

This describes dysfunction of the urinary bladder due to disease of the central or peripheral nervous system involved in the control of micturition.

Micturition depends on the integration of neuronal pathways between the cerebral cortex, brainstem and sacral spinal cord. Therefore, causes of a neurogenic bladder encompass both traumatic and atraumatic insults at varying levels, including the cerebral cortex and spinal cord. Those that affect the spinal cord above the sacral level produce an upper motor neuron pattern of injury. Insults at the level of the sacrum and lower result in a lower motor neuron deficit.

When evaluating the effect of a spinal cord injury (SCI) on bladder function, consider the level affected, as this alters the clinical presentation and will guide bladder management (*Table 6.1*). This is particularly important in supra-sacral spinal cord level injuries where urgent intervention may be required for a high-pressure urinary tract in order to protect renal function. The primary concern for long-term management of the neurogenic bladder is to preserve kidney function, and secondarily, to treat symptomatic lower urinary tract symptoms.

Note that patients with complete or partial SCI at the same level can present differently. Also, patients can have defects at multiple levels (such as in multiple

Table 6.1 Neurological problems and their effect on the urinary tract.

Level of lesion	Example of neurological problem	Effect on the urinary tract
Brain (supra-pontine)	Parkinson's disease, stroke, MS, tumours, dementia	Discoordination/inappropriate voiding Bladder overactivity (Safe, low-pressure bladder)
Supra-sacral spinal cord (between the pons and L5 level)	SCI, spina bifida, disc prolapse (upper motor neuron pattern of injury)	Overactive bladder/detrusor hyperreflexia DSD Stiffer bladder (poor compliance) (Dangerous bladder; high pressure, risk to kidneys)
Conus (sacral spinal cord from S1 to S5 or peripheral nerves)	Cauda equina, SCI, peripheral neuropathy (including causes such as diabetes) (lower motor neuron pattern of injury)	Underactive bladder (urinary retention) Detrusor areflexia Weak external urethral sphincter (causing incontinence) (Safe, low-pressure bladder)

DSD: detrusor sphincter dyssynergia; MS: multiple sclerosis; SCI: spinal cord injury.

sclerosis), and clinical presentation may be variable.

Urological emergencies that may present to the emergency department in patients with underlying neurological causes include the following as outlined below.

Autonomic dysreflexia

This is a significant acute medical emergency characterised by severe uncontrolled peripheral hypertension, which can occur in patients with SCI at or above the level of the 6th thoracic vertebrae (T6). A significant sensory stimulus entering the spinal cord via intact peripheral nerves induces a large sympathetic output from thoracolumbar sympathetic nerves, resulting in widespread vasoconstriction (particularly splanchnic vascular bed). Due to the level of injury, descending inhibitory impulses are unable to exert an effect at sympathetic outflow sites, and compensatory increased parasympathetic vagal cardiac input (bradycardia) is inadequate, thereby uncontrolled peripheral arterial hypertension ensues.

The stimulus is usually bladder or bowel in origin. Urological triggers include bladder distension (**Figure 6.5**), urinary tract calculus, urological intervention (such as catheterisation or cystoscopy) and UTI.

Complications of stroke, seizure, cardiac complications and death can occur if autonomic dysreflexia is left unresolved.

Presentation
A high index of suspicion is required and you should look out for the following features:

* Symptoms:
  › Profuse sweating around the face and neck.
  › Nasal congestion.
  › Blurred vision.
  › Headache.
  › Anxiety.

* Signs:
  › Rise in systolic and diastolic blood pressure (BP) above baseline (note BP baseline is often low in spinal cord injury).
  › Bradycardia.
  › Pupil constriction.
  › Skin changes above the level of the lesion = parasympathetic responses: flushing and sweating.
  › Skin changes below the level of the lesion = sympathetic responses: pale, cool skin with piloerection.

Management
* Sit the patient upright (and loosen tight clothing or belts).
* Examine for a distended bladder and treat.
* If a catheter is present, ensure it is draining. If it is blocked, change the catheter.
* Perform a rectal exam to exclude faecal impaction as a cause.
* Ensure BP is monitored; a short-acting antihypertensive may be indicated for BP control, but this will not resolve a hypertensive crisis if the underlying stimulus is not removed.

Cauda equina
This is caused by compression on the spinal roots. It can be due to benign causes such as lumbar disc rupture, spinal infection, spinal fracture, spinal haematoma, spinal canal stenosis, blunt and penetrating spinal trauma or arteriovenous malformation. Malignant causes include spinal cord tumours or metastases – this is covered in full on pages 125–126. Patients present acutely with lower back pain, lower limb weakness and numbness, and

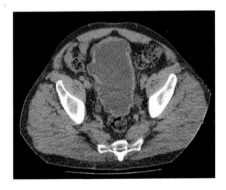

Figure 6.5 Axial pelvic CT image of a high-pressure 'unsafe' neuropathic bladder. Note multiple bladder diverticulae, a thickened bladder wall and bilaterally dilated distal ureters. These appearances are sometimes referred to as a 'fir-tree' or 'pine cone' bladder.

sudden-onset bladder, bowel and sexual dysfunction. An emergency magnetic resonance imaging (MRI) of the spine is required. If the diagnosis is confirmed, steroids and decompressive surgery to relieve pressure on the nerves is required urgently, under the care of spinal or neurological surgeons. Antibiotics are given for any infective processes.

Acute spinal cord injury

This can be caused by blunt or penetrating trauma resulting in injury to the spinal vertebrae, discs or ligaments of the vertebral column or to the spinal cord directly, and can be complicated by haematoma. Injuries can be complete or incomplete, and the manifestations on the urinary tract will depend on the level of the injury and nerves directly affected (motor, sensory and autonomic nerves can be involved).

Spinal shock is the sudden loss of spinal reflex activity below the level of the SCI. This causes passive bladder filling and subsequent overflow incontinence. The duration of this areflexia depends on the level of the lesion. It may last weeks, particularly if the injury affects sacral segments causing a sacral areflexia, typified by flaccid paraplegia, reduced anal tone and loss of sensation in the sacral dermatomes. Awareness of this can allow prompt catheter insertion that will form the basis of acute management.

Management

An urethral indwelling catheter should be inserted immediately for the acute phase of resuscitation and to mitigate the problem of passive bladder filling causing distension in spinal shock. Care should be taken to prevent traction on the catheter with placement of a catheter restrainer. Once the spinal injury is stable, aim for removal of the indwelling catheter and start clean intermittent self-catheterisation (CISC) if required. A suprapubic catheter can be used when patients cannot perform CISC.

Assessment of other general problems relating to the urinary tract in neuropathic patients

History

- Clarify the underlying neurological disorder or injury and at what level the spinal cord is affected.
- How does the condition affect other organs (e.g. bowel incontinence, sexual dysfunction, mobility, manual dexterity)?
- Is the neurological problem stable or progressive?
  - › Stable – SCI, spina bifida.
  - › Progressive – stroke, multiple sclerosis, Parkinson's disease.
- Any previous urinary tract surgery? (Patients with long-term conditions such as spina bifida may have had several operations already for bladder problems or incontinence).
- Is there new disruption to storage and/ or emptying of the bladder?
- Drug and treatment history – is the patient on any drugs that might affect their bladder function (i.e. anticholinergic medication is used for an overactive bladder, but has a risk of urinary retention)?

Examination

- Inspection – the patient may have scars from previous neurological surgery relating to their neurological problems or complications associated with their condition which they may not have told you about (ventriculoperitoneal shunt, Mitrofanoff, colostomy).

- Standard examination of the abdomen, perineum with vaginal or rectal examination, assessing for a palpable bladder, prolapse, an enlarged or suspicious prostate.
- Neurological assessment, including assessment of the lower limbs, back and rectal examination to establish if there is normal peri-anal sensation and anal tone (where clinically appropriate). Be vigilant for signs of an undiagnosed neurological disorder (i.e. sacral agenesis, spina bifida occulta).

Investigation

- Urinalysis and culture: to assess for infection. Proteinuria and haematuria may also be an indicator of renal impairment, and requires further assessment.
- Bloods, including urea and creatinine for renal function testing.
- USS KUB to assess for any evidence of upper tract obstruction and to assess if the bladder empties adequately. If patients have high-pressure bladders or if they retain urine (chronic retention) they are at risk of upper tract dilatation and renal deterioration.
- Appropriate neurological imaging dependent on first or recurrent presentation of neurological sequelae. If the patient presents acutely with new-onset lower limb weakness and urinary retention, an MRI of the spine is required to rule out spinal cord or cauda equina compression or injury.

- Urodynamic studies may be offered in the outpatient setting.

Management

Treatment decisions will depend on neurological aetiology, whether the neurological disorder is stable or progressive, its effect on associated organ function and the individual patient's wishes. The main aims to achieve are outlined below.

Protection of the upper renal tracts:

- Overactive bladder – reduce pressure in the bladder by CISC. Alternative interventions include:
  › Bladder augmentation – using a bowel patch to relieve the pressure build up, e.g. clam ileocystoplasty.
  › Disruption of micturition reflex arc – via dorsal rhizotomy (dorsal sacral nerve roots surgically divided) with implantation of a sacral root stimulator.
  › Botulinum toxin (botox) – injected intravesically to relax the muscle of the bladder, which increases its capacity and lowers its pressure.
  › Sacral root neuromodulation – achieved via implantation of an S3 sacral root stimulator.
  › Urinary diversion – formation of an ileal conduit for refractory cases.
- Chronic retention – may require a catheter (often suprapubic) if urodynamic studies reveal a high-pressure bladder. CISC is preferable to an indwelling catheter if the patient has appropriate manual

dexterity and cognitive function, as there is a lower risk of UTI.

- Detrusor sphincter dyssynergia (DSD) – this is discoordinated synchronous contraction of both the bladder and urethral sphincter at the same time, which causes problems passing urine and can lead to high pressures in the bladder (which can be transmitted to the upper tracts). This can be treated with regular CISC or the use of catheters, injection of botox into the external sphincter, surgical division of the external sphincter or sacral nerve neuromodulation.

Management of stress incontinence (i.e. due to sphincter weakness).
Conservative management options include an indwelling catheter or using a condom sheath drainage device, e.g. Conveen®, in males. Surgical management in women includes: urethral bulking agents, mid-urethral tapes, pubovaginal slings and colposuspension. Insertion of an artificial urinary sphincter can be offered to both women and men. Bladder neck closure can be performed in intractable cases, but will require formation of a catheterisable continent channel (such as a Mitrofanoff) to drain the bladder via an alternative route. Finally, urinary diversion with an ileal conduit could be considered.

Prevention of recurrent lower urinary tract infections
Address any chronic retention, and treat any reversible causes for UTIs. Prophylactic low-dose antibiotics are sometimes considered (see page 63).

Key Points

- Be aware of the risk of autonomic dysreflexia in spinal cord injuries at or above T6 and treat triggers such as a distended bladder quickly.

- Cauda equina compression manifests with urinary retention along with back pain and lower limb weakness, and needs an urgent MRI, steroids and spinal decompression surgery.

- After spinal cord injury, there is a period of spinal shock that can cause bladder dysfunction – so catheterise the bladder in the early stages.

- In cases of neurogenic bladder, protection of the upper urinary tracts is a priority, whilst minimising infection risk

ONCOLOGICAL EMERGENCIES[4]

Although urological (and non-urological) cancers are encountered in everyday urological practice, there are certain emergency situations where timely diagnosis and management can significantly affect outcome.

Malignant spinal cord compression

Threatened or actual neurological disability can be caused by local extension of malignancy or metastasis causing pressure (either directly or by vertebral collapse) on the spinal cord or cauda equina (**Figure 6.6**).

Metastatic spinal cord compression (MSCC) is an oncological emergency such that if recognition and management of it is delayed it can worsen neurological sequelae and can result in permanent paraplegia.

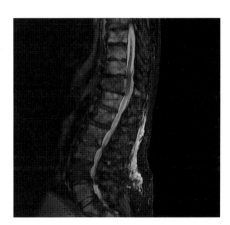

Figure 6.6 Sagittal STIR MRI image demonstrating widespread bony metastases and metastatic epidural mass causing narrowing of the spinal canal and cord compression at the level of T11. (Image courtesy of Dr J. Libiszewski.)

Not all cases will be due to a urological cancer, but being able to recognise how it presents and what needs to be done next is important. Also, be aware that some patients presenting with spinal cord metastases have no prior diagnosis of cancer. Prostate cancer can spread to the bones, and so prostate cancer patients with metastatic disease are at risk of MSCC.

History
- Presenting features:
  › Back pain – particularly thoracic as this is the region most frequently affected by MSCC, but also any severe, progressive or unremitting spinal pain is possible with reports that the pain is often worse at night.
  › Radicular pain (pain that radiates into the lower extremity along the course of a spinal nerve root).
  › Limb weakness or difficulty walking.
  › Sensory loss.
  › Bladder or bowel dysfunction (including urinary retention and incontinence).
  › Sudden onset sexual dysfunction.
- Past medical history:
  › Any known malignancy or metastatic disease.
  › Background lower urinary tract symptoms, which may have deteriorated suddenly.

Examination
- Assess for localised spine tenderness, and try to establish the sensory level on neurological examination.
- Lower motor neuron signs at the level of the lesion, i.e. atrophy, hyporeflexia.
- Upper motor neuron lesions below that level, i.e. upgoing plantar reflex, hyperreflexia, clonus, spasticity.

- Cauda equina syndrome occurs if there is compression of the cauda equina below the level of L2.
- Anal sphincter tone reduced; reduced peri-anal sensation.
- Digital rectal exam to check for prostate malignancy.

Investigation
- Bloods (including FBC, urea and electrolytes [U&E] and liver function tests to look for potential bone marrow depletion, renal obstruction and liver involvement from metastatic disease) and most recent prostate-specific antigen (PSA). Note, the PSA levels can be artificially elevated following catheterisation or urethral instrumentation. It is rare to have metastatic bone disease from prostate cancer if the PSA is <20ng/ml.
- MRI of the whole spine – The National Institute for Health and Care Excellence (NICE) guidelines state that this should be performed to allow for definitive treatment to be planned within 1 week in the case of spinal pain suggestive of spinal metastases, and within 24 hours if there are additional neurological signs or symptoms of MSCC, including out-of-hours investigation for emergency treatment (thus may require hospital transfer)[1].

Management
- Nurse the patient lying flat with neutral spine alignment until neurological/spinal stability is confirmed.
- Liaise with the oncology team early.
- Initiate a course of dexamethasone – at least 16mg after assessment, then a 16mg daily short course – whilst

definitive treatment is being planned (unless contraindicated).
- Catheterise for bladder dysfunction.
- Pain control: adequate analgesia initially.
- Palliative radiotherapy, spinal orthoses and spine stabilisation surgery should be considered.
- Offer bisphosphonates to patients with prostate cancer if analgesia is not effective.
- If deemed appropriate, definitive treatment, e.g. radiotherapy or surgery, should be arranged before further neurological deterioration and within 24 hours of diagnosis of spinal cord compression.
- Venous thromboembolism (VTE) assessment and monitoring for pressure sores.
- Well-documented and ongoing discussion with the patient regarding their treatment wishes should be a priority.

Bilateral malignant ureteric obstruction

Both urological and non-urological cancers can obstruct the ureteric orifices. As such, it may be that the patient presents with renal failure with a known urological cancer, or this may be picked up on a scan arranged by another team who seek advice from urology. If asymptomatic, unilateral ureteric obstruction (and the presence of a normal contralateral kidney) picked up incidentally may simply warrant urgent outpatient investigation. Bilateral ureteric obstruction, on the other hand, demands emergency urological intervention.

History
- Patients may notice reduced urinary

output (oliguria or anuria), with associated symptoms of renal failure (i.e. fluid retention, shortness of breath, drowsiness, nausea, confusion, itching).

- Ask about any previous cancer diagnosis (prostate, ureteric, bladder, cervical, renal, lymphoma) and the treatment they have already received to date.

Examination

- General constitution.
- Abdominal exam – scars of previous cancer surgery; examine for masses; bladder likely not palpable.
- Rectal (PR) or vaginal (PV) exam to examine for masses.

Investigation

- Bloods including renal function and clotting (required before consideration of nephrostomy).
- A bladder scan will show an empty bladder (unless there is a significant tumour burden).
- USS KUB will show hydronephrosis (unilateral or bilateral).

Management

- Treatment of electrolyte abnormalities, e.g. hyperkalaemia.
- Immediate intervention for bilateral upper tract obstruction will need discussion with interventional radiology colleagues (and likely involvement of the urology team) for an emergency procedure – bilateral nephrostomies or percutaneous renal puncture and placement of ureteric stents (antegrade, i.e. through the kidney, as opposed to retrograde from the bladder, as the tumour is likely to be obscuring the ureteric orifices within the bladder). Both methods allow drainage of the kidneys but both have their advantages and disadvantages. Nephrostomy tubes allow definite drainage of both kidneys but the patient is left with two urine collection bags and possible repeat trips with nephrostomy complications and replacements. Ureteric stents allow internal drainage but can themselves become blocked from extrinsic compression. Retrograde stents generally require general anaesthesia for insertion, which may come with increased risks in a patient with renal compromise and malignant disease. Hence, given both options have problems, careful counselling needs to occur, as some patients, when faced with these options, may decline further life-prolonging treatment. Some patients in this situation (where their underlying malignancy may have a poor prognosis) may elect to accept stents for palliation of symptoms associated with the obstruction.

- Long-term treatment options vary but should be decided taking into account the patient's prognosis and wishes.

POST-OPERATIVE EMERGENCIES[5]

With almost a quarter of a million urological procedures performed per year in the UK, urology as a specialty treats a large number of patients. While most follow a straightforward and predictable post-operative course, it is important to be aware that complications can occur, and when they do, recognise them quickly and deal with them appropriately. With such a wide range of interventions, from minor day-case procedures through to large, life-changing and life-saving operations, the range of complications is varied. Here we outline some of the common emergencies seen post-operatively, both during the hospital stay, and after the patient is discharged to the community. An awareness, not only of these common post-operative complications, but also of the operation itself is important in anticipation and early recognition of complications. If at all possible, look at the original operation notes, paying particular attention to the estimated blood loss, irrigation volume required and any comment on final haemostasis.

In the unwell patient, the initial management is always to resuscitate the patient (ABCDE) and call for help where needed.

Inpatient post-operative complications

Bleeding/haematuria

Haematuria may be seen after a range of urological procedures, but details are given below firstly on stone surgery where, rarely, bleeding can be serious and related to the kidney and, secondly, on commonly performed procedures such as prostate surgery:

- Percutaneous nephrolithotomy (PCNL) – 'taking stones out of the kidney' and 'through the skin' – an operation used to remove large renal stones percutaneously. A nephrostomy drain is often left at the end of the procedure.

- Ureteroscopic stone fragmentation/ removal – endoscopic removal of stones from the ureter or kidney using an instrument inserted typically via the urethra and bladder.
- Extracorporeal shock wave lithotripsy (ESWL) – 'breaking up stones by ultrasonic shockwaves' and 'from outside of the body'. Ultrasound or fluoroscopy are used to locate a stone in the kidney or ureter, and an acoustic shockwave is directed at the stone (from outside the body) to fragment the stone.

Haematuria after stone surgery occurs in most cases and is of little significance when self-limiting and lasting less than 24 hours. Rarely, bleeding complications can be more serious, including perinephric and renal haematomas. The bleeding risk associated with PCNL is much higher than with ESWL. Significant bleeding should be suspected in patients with pre-existing anticoagulant or antiplatelet therapy, abdominal pain and haemodynamic instability. Important points in the management of bleeding following stone surgery are listed below, followed by an approach to significant haematuria following TURP:

- Remember to look at the operation note for procedural details.
- Full examination to assess fluid volume status and for any abdominal pain/ renal angle bruising or tenderness.
- Monitor the patient for a drop in haemoglobin or blood pressure as well as tachycardia – if any of these occurs, consider organising an urgent CT angiography to look for active bleeding.
- Patients who have undergone

PCNL may be left with a draining nephrostomy. Look at the drainage fluid type and volume. If there is evidence of heavy bleeding into the nephrostomy bag, the first management is to clamp the nephrostomy to achieve tamponade of the bleeding, followed by further radiological investigation and definitive treatment.

- Generally, where active bleeding is identified on imaging or is apparent clinically, patients need embolisation by interventional radiology in the first instance (**Figure 6.7**). Rarely, surgery is indicated.

Bleeding after endoscopic bladder outlet surgery is common. For this reason many surgeons will leave a 3-way catheter *in situ* post-operatively. Monopolar transurethral resection of the prostate (TURP) may be associated with the most bleeding, but the following could be used if haematuria fails to settle after alternative procedures (e.g. HoLEP):

- Additional water can be added to the catheter balloon (add a further 20–30ml after making sure that the catheter is pushed back to the bladder) and gentle traction can be applied to the catheter. The catheter balloon tends to fall into the prostatic fossa and exerts haemostatic pressure, therefore helping to tamponade bleeding. Typical silicone 3-way catheter balloons can hold up to 50ml of water but always check the markings on the fluid port. Initial teaching would suggest traction should not occur for more than 1 hour, but there is no evidence to support this and the author has

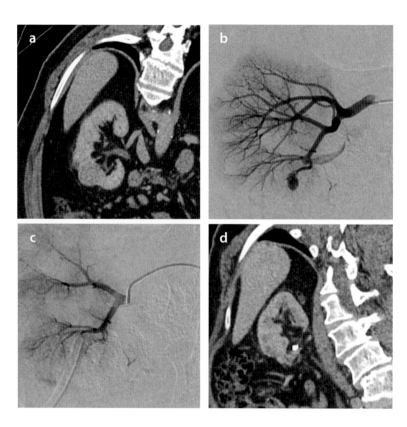

Figure 6.7 Partial nephrectomy bleed. Coronal CT of the right kidney (**a**) showing a lower pole renal cell carcinoma. Digital subtraction angiogram (**b**) showing a small pseudoaneurysm at the site of the partial nephrectomy as the cause of the post-operative haematuria. Digital subtraction angiogram (**c**) following coil embolisation sealing the pseudoaneurysm. Coronal CT image (**d**) showing preservation of the upper pole of the kidney with an embolisation coil and partial nephrectomy scar at the lower pole.

used overnight traction when needed. Short-term immediate traction is best performed with an individual doctor pulling on the catheter, but longer-term traction can be applied by tying a weight (such as a saline irrigation bag) to the catheter and hanging this over the end of the bed.

Catheter falls out after surgery

Sometimes a catheter falling out is merely inconvenient, and would not qualify as an emergency so long as the patient is able to pass urine. However, in some circumstances, urgent replacement of a catheter is indicated as discussed below:

- TURP:
  › After TURP a 20–24 Fr 3-way catheter is placed (with balloon inflated to at least 20ml) to allow irrigation for 12–24 hours.
  › Positioning of the catheter balloon in the prostatic fossa provides haemostatic pressure, thus if the catheter falls out soon after surgery, it should be replaced as in the above specification to help to reduce the risk of immediate post-operative bleeding and urinary retention. If the patient is 1–2 days post-operative, and the urine is clear or a light rose pink colour, it is reasonable not to replace the catheter and have a trial of voiding instead.
- Radical prostatectomy (open, laparoscopic or robotic):
  › Post-operatively, the catheter usually remains in place for 1 week to allow for healing at the bladder neck and urethral anastomosis. If it falls out, reinsertion should be performed by a senior urologist to avoid inadvertent damage to the urinary tract and breakdown of the new anastomosis.
  › Recatheterisation in this situation is safest when performed under cystoscopic guidance, usually by flexible cystoscopy under local anaesthetic.

An emergency situation may also arise when a catheter falls out as a result of the patient pulling it out themselves, commonly due to delirium or dementia. In this instance it would be prudent to examine the patient to assess for trauma to the urethra, but also the catheter itself, to assess the likelihood of retention of a catheter fragment in the bladder. If this is suspected, a cystoscopic removal of the fragment may be required. Judgement is then required as to whether the catheter needs replacing on an urgent basis, taking into account the indication for catheterisation and how appropriate it would be to replace the catheter if the patient is distressed (consider the issue of consent).

TUR syndrome

TUR syndrome refers to a dilutional hyponatraemia secondary to absorption of large volumes of bladder irrigant. There can also be an associated glycine toxicity if glycine irrigation is used.

TUR syndrome can occur in any procedure using large volumes of irrigation (bladder, prostate or renal surgery); however, it is most commonly described with glycine irrigation for transurethral resection of the prostate. The risk increases with longer procedures, significant bleeding, or if the prostate capsule is breached opening the venous plexuses. It can also occur if prolonged saline irrigation is used. It can manifest peri- or post-operatively.

The patient can develop hypertension, bradycardia, nausea and vomiting, confusion, visual disturbance (flashing lights), bradycardia and seizures.

Initial management involves fluid restriction and slowing the rate of bladder irrigation; check renal function/sodium levels.

The patient should be managed in a high-care facility with very close monitoring of fluid balance.

Correction of hyponatraemia with hypertonic saline or furosemide and general supportive medical measures may be required.

Anuria/oliguria (normal adult urine output = 0.5ml/kg/h)

It is important to distinguish between pre-renal, renal and post-renal causes of renal dysfunction (see AKI, Chapter 2); however, if the patient is euvolaemic (appropriately hydrated), non-responsive to fluid challenges and there is no obvious factor that could cause intrinsic renal damage, it follows that with instrumentation of the urinary tract or previous urological history, the likely cause is post-renal. A useful guide to assessing the cause of post-renal/obstructive causes is based on anatomical level:

- Obstruction at the level of the bladder/bladder outlet:
  › Is there a catheter *in situ*? If yes, is it draining at all? Can it be flushed using sterile irrigation fluid and a bladder syringe? If no, is there a palpable bladder/evidence of urinary retention on a bladder scan? If so, insert a urinary catheter and monitor urine output.
  › Has there been recent radical prostate surgery that formed a bladder neck anastomosis? For example, in radical prostatectomy, if there is a leak at the urethra–bladder anastomosis, urine will leak intraperitoneally, causing a chemical peritonitis. It is very important to ensure that the catheter is *in situ* and draining in this scenario.

- At the level of the ureteric orifices or ureters:
  › Is there known bladder cancer/recent TURBT? Is there any locally advanced cancer that could cause bilateral ureteric obstruction? (See the section on oncological emergencies.)
  Check the cystoscopy operation notes – were the ureteric orifices visible and preserved?
  Check recent imaging – could the tumour burden involve the ureteric orifices or compress the ureters?
  › Are both kidneys known to function normally? If not, what could obstruct the ureter draining the previously functioning kidney, e.g. passage of ureteric calculi or post ESWL collection of fragments in the ureter ('steinstrasse'). Remember the obstruction may be anywhere along the ureter, from where it enters the bladder (vesicoureteric junction) to where it drains the renal pelvis (pelviureteric junction).

Post-catheterisation diuresis

This is most commonly seen after catheterisation in chronic urinary retention, but can occur after relief of obstruction at any level in the urinary system (see also pages 49–50). The risk is greater if:

- There is a high residual volume of urine drained initially.
- There is evidence of renal impairment.

Those at increased risk will need observation of urine output. The key things to do when asked to catheterise, in order to help decide whether admission is required are:

- Perform a bladder scan prior to catheterisation to anticipate how large a volume is likely to drain.
- Document the volume of urine drained after the initial 5–10 minutes from catheter insertion and document this as the residual volume.
- Ensure bloods are taken to check renal function (as early as possible so the results are available to make a decision).

If patients are at high risk for diuresis as described above, then they should be monitored closely with:

- Accurate documentation of hourly urine output and monitor vital signs.
- Clear instructions to nursing colleagues regarding fluid volume replacement: an example of this may be "after initial 4 hours, if urine output exceeds 200ml/h, give IV fluids at a rate that replaces half of the hourly volume of urine lost".
- Daily U&E if there is evidence of diuresis to check for electrolyte abnormalities

and renal function. Beware of the risk of hypokalaemia despite common high potassium levels at presentation.
- Lying and standing blood pressure and daily weights to assess fluid replacement is adequate.

Compartment syndrome

Compartment syndrome is ischaemia to muscles and nerves due to tissue pressure within a closed compartment exceeding perfusion pressure.

Compartment syndrome should not be forgotten in urology. The condition is not uncommon in the lower limbs with its risk increased in prolonged procedures with pressure on muscle compartments, for example in the lithotomy position.

- Have a high index of suspicion if the patient reports unremitting pain or pain out of proportion, and pain on passive stretch of muscle compartments.
- Do not wait for neurovascular compromise (paraesthesia, cool peripheries) to act on suspicion.
- Compartment syndrome can cause rhabdomyolysis and renal failure – needs urgent intervention in the form of fasciotomies to preserve tissue and ultimately protect the kidneys.

Urinary tract infection and sepsis

- Genitourinary tract intervention, instrumentation or surgery is associated with a risk of urinary infection or sepsis. Urine is checked at pre-assessment, and also on the day of surgery in selected patients to avoid proceeding with surgery in patients with active untreated UTI. Local microbiology (and the European

Association of Urology) guidelines provide information on the best antibiotic prophylaxis to be given at induction.

- If a patient shows evidence of infection or sepsis post-surgery, check the operation notes and see whether any antibiotics were given to cover the procedure. Culture blood and urine. Request microbiology advice about the best empirical antibiotics to give whilst waiting for definitive sensitivities.

- The presence of any prostheses in the urinary tract can act as a nidus of infection or harbour infection, which makes it difficult to eradicate the source of infection (i.e. testicular prosthesis, artificial urinary sphincter, mesh tape for stress incontinence surgery). If infection fails to respond to appropriate antibiotics, the prosthetic device needs to be removed.

- As in any post-operative course, urgent assessment and treatment should be instigated if sepsis is suspected (see Chapter 1, pages 12-15). Initial management is with resuscitation. Treat any reversible causes.

Outpatient post-operative complications

Bleeding/haematuria
- Primary bleeding following prostate or bladder tumour resection (TURP/TURBT) will often manifest itself as visible haematuria or clot retention seen peri-operatively and continuing in the early post-operative recovery period.
- Secondary bleeding usually occurs at day 10–14, due to haemostatic

'scabs' of healing tissue falling away. In mild cases of haematuria with haemodynamic stability and no associated voiding problems, advice and encouragement to maintain a good fluid intake may be all that is required, with antibiotics if there is any sign of infection.

- Severe bleeding and/or difficulty passing urine and concerns of clot passage or retention will need assessment in hospital:
  › Examination to assess volume status.
  › Check FBC, renal function and inflammatory markers.
  › If there is evidence of haematuria with clots, insert a 20–24 Fr 3-way catheter and perform a bladder washout to remove any existing clots. Set up continuous irrigation if clots are detected to prevent further clot formation.
  › If the patient is haemodynamically compromised and/or heavy bleeding persists, the patient may require a return to theatre or radiological intervention (angiography +/- embolisation).

Poor cosmesis and concerns after day-case procedures
- Hydrocoele repair: a degree of discomfort and swelling is common after hydrocoele repair. The patient should be carefully counselled before surgery. A scrotal support or scrotal elevation can help this. Patients are also informed of the chance of permanent 'lumpiness' behind the testicle at the surgical site. If there is significant swelling in the post-operative course, the patient may need

reviewing to distinguish between haematoma formation and surgical site infection, which can require surgical drainage. Assessment should take into consideration the time elapsed since surgery, degree of swelling and whether there is evidence of systemic or local signs of infection. Ultrasound of the scrotum can help assess for signs of haematoma or abscess.

- Circumcision: patients are told to expect 3–4 days of swelling at the operation site. They may well seek medical attention if they have a temperature, or notice increased swelling, redness or discharge at the surgical site. In this case they will need reviewing for wound breakdown and surgical site infection. This should be distinguished from poor cosmetic outcome, which may need a follow-up urology opinion, but does not require an emergency urology assessment. A circumcised penis can take up to 6 weeks to heal fully, and will look very unsightly for at least 2 weeks.

- Vasectomy: haematoma in a post-vasectomy procedure for male contraception may occur. Depending on the degree of the swelling and progressive increase in size or infection (fluctuant mass, increased warmth, redness or pyrexia), USS should be considered to look for infected haematoma. In most cases conservative management with or without antibiotics is sufficient, but in cases where there are concerns of active bleeding or abscess formation, surgical exploration may be indicated. The patient needs to be warned of an increased risk of failure as a result of recanalisation of the vas deferens due to an infective process.

Key Points

- The approach to an unwell post-operative patient should combine diagnosis and resuscitation.

- With unstable patients, escalate early and call for senior help.

- Refer back to the operation notes whenever assessing complications following urological surgery.

- TUR syndrome can occur after any prolonged transurethral procedure. Prolonged surgery, significant intra-operative bleeding, use of glycine irrigation and breach of the protastic capsule all increase the risk.

- Should the urethral catheter fall out soon after a radical prostatectomy (robotic, laparoscopic or open) reinsertion should be performed by a senior urologist, often using cystoscopy.

TUBES, PROSTHESES AND ALTERED URINARY TRACT ANATOMY[6]

When urine cannot drain freely through the renal system, there is a risk of damage to the kidneys – a post-renal (obstructive) kidney injury.

It is usually possible to determine the anatomical location at which there is an obstruction to urinary flow. We will look at how 'tubes', in the form of ureteric stents or nephrostomies, can allow drainage of the kidneys. Conversely, if there is impedance to bladder outflow and urethral catheterisation is not possible, a catheter can be sited suprapubically to allow the bladder to drain. We will also consider the use of devices and prostheses in urology, and how various types of urological surgery modify native anatomy, focusing on how to deal with acute issues related to this altered anatomy.

Ureteric stents

Stents are thin plastic tubes inserted into one or both ureters either via cystoscopy from the bladder (retrograde access) or percutaneously through the kidney (antegrade access), which requires radio-logical guidance. They are called 'JJ' stents or 'pigtail' stents as they curl at either end once inserted to help maintain their position. They are available in different lengths and diameters – 6 Fr polymer stents are the most commonly used stents in adult patients, ranging from 22–30cm in length.

Stents are used to decompress the ureter when there is an intrinsic blockage (such as a stone or clot). They are used electively following ureteroscopy and laser fragmentation of ureteric stones as a prophylactic measure to reduce the risk of obstruction due to ureteric oedema, (and later removed). They are also used for cases of external compression of the ureters, seen in retroperitoneal fibrosis, or with pelvic tumours, pelvic collections or lymphadenopathy.

If they need to remain *in situ*, they usually need changing every 6 months; however, most are licensed for 12-month use. In pregnancy, this must be reduced to every 4–6 weeks as stent encrustation is accelerated.

If a patient presents with problems potentially relating to the presence of a ureteric stent, check renal function, inflammatory markers and ensure urine samples are sent for culture. An abdominal X-ray can help assess stent location +/- USS KUB or CTKUB to assess stent position more accurately and for new hydronephrosis. Common problems related to indwelling ureteric stents are listed below.

Problems
- Pain: the patient is counselled to expect a certain degree of stent-related pain prior to their insertion but may need to investigate further for complications of stent insertion such as infection and migration/displacement. There is some evidence that tamsulosin (400µg OD) may reduce stent-related pain.
- Stent migration/displacement: may present with pain but also a change in urine output. The stent position can be checked with a KUB X-ray (**Figure 6.8**), USS or CT scan. A displaced stent may need replacement or removal.
- Lower urinary tract symptoms: as there is a curl of plastic stent sitting in the bladder, it is common that patients report urinary frequency, urgency and

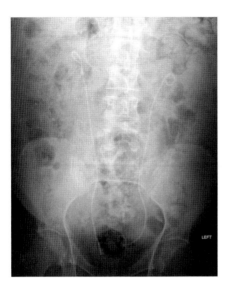

Figure 6.8 Plain abdominal radiograph demonstrating bilateral ureteric JJ stents in normal positions. A coil in the stent should be visible at both ends, corresponding to the renal pelvis and the urinary bladder.

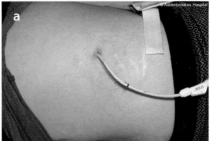

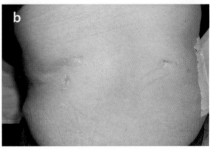

Figure 6.9 (a) Right-sided nephrostomy, with overlying dressings removed viewed from the patient's side; (b) scars on both flanks demonstrate previous nephrostomy sites. Note how posteriorly nephrostomy tubes are often sited, necessitating examination of the back of a patient.

even incontinence in women. Only if the patient has systemic symptoms of a UTI with positive urinalysis should they be considered in the category of a complicated UTI, and treated with antibiotics.

Nephrostomy tubes

A nephrostomy is a thin plastic tube inserted percutaneously into the kidney (through the renal parenchyma to sit in the renal pelvis) under ultrasound or fluoroscopy guidance (**Figure 6.9**). It has a single pigtail or coil that helps to retain the device in the kidney. It is also secured to the skin with an adhesive dressing and

clip appliance. The urine drains from the kidney out of the tubing into a collection bag, which is strapped to the leg, with a tap to empty the bag once full.

A nephrostomy tube allows relief of pressure and drainage of the kidney, thereby protecting it from obstructive damage. It allows urinary drainage when the ureter is obstructed and retrograde access (via the ureter) is not possible or is unsafe. This may be in the context of an infected obstructed kidney due to a calculus, obstructive tumour growth (e.g. advanced prostate cancer or retroperitoneal tumours such as ovarian) compressing the ureters (and where ureteric stents may fail to achieve adequate drainage) or if other mechanical abnormalities prevent drainage.

The drainage bag needs changing weekly. The nephrostomy tube itself is usually changed at 3 months initially, then at 6-month intervals thereafter in the radiology department under a local anaesthetic.

Problems
- Not draining:
  - › Check the tubing is not kinked and no mechanical obstruction exists.
  - › Flush using an aseptic technique. Open a sterile dressing pack and prepare 5–10ml sterile normal saline in a syringe. Using an aseptic technique, disconnect the drainage system from the main nephrostomy tubing and flush the nephrostomy gently with 10ml aliquots of normal saline (this can be repeated if required).
  - › Allow urine/saline to flow out of the tube.
  - › If not draining or there is a difficulty in flushing, try gentle aspiration. If nothing will go in or come out of the nephrostomy tubing, it may be displaced, and require a nephrostogram +/- reinsertion in the radiology department.
  - › Apply a new bag if the system is now draining freely.
- Fallen out/dislodged/leaking:
  - › It may be apparent that the tube has entirely come out/broken off or this may present as the tube not draining, as described above. Remember to examine for any leakage at the nephrostomy site.
  - › If the tube is not draining or is visibly dislodged, then contact the urology on-call for advice.

In the meantime, take bloods to check renal function, clotting profile and FBC. The nephrostomy will require replacement in the radiology department. They will usually use the old track if access with a guidewire is possible; if not, a new tract will need to be made, so clotting is checked to ensure it is normal. If the patient is on anticoagulation, this will need to be stopped, and in some cases, the effects reversed (in an emergency) to allow nephrostomy insertion (if a ureteric stent is not possible).

- Dressing needs changing and/or nephrostomy site is inflamed/infected:
  - › This is done under aseptic technique so ensure you have a dressing pack, saline solution, gauze and sterile adhesive dressings.
  - › Remove the old dressing carefully without pulling out the nephrostomy tube (which may be sutured to the skin).
  - › Swab for a culture if the area looks infected or a discharge is visible.
  - › Clean the area around the tube with saline, then allow to dry before replacing gauze folded up once either side of the tube, and securing with Tegaderm™ or similar adhesive dressing.
  - › Use another Tegaderm™ to secure the tubing to the patient's skin to avoid pulling out.

At the bottom of the tube there is a white clip with a piece of thread hanging from it (**Figure 6.10**). The black thread, when under tension produces the pigtail curve in the nephrostomy tubing placed within the kidney. To remove a nephrostomy, this thread needs to be released and cut in order to allow the nephrostomy tip to uncurl. Attempts to remove the nephrostomy without releasing the thread can lead to renal trauma. Nephrostomies should sometimes be removed under fluoroscopy guidance in the radiology department. Decisions to remove a nephrostomy should always be discussed with the urology team.

- UTI/temperature:
    - › A UTI in the context of an indwelling urological device such as a nephrostomy tube is by definition a complicated UTI.
    - › In such an instance, systemic signs such as fever with or without localised urinary symptoms may represent a symptomatic UTI that requires treatment.
    - › With indwelling urological devices, there may be chronic bacteriuria, but that does not mean that you

should not take a urine sample. A urine sample should still always be sent for culture and sensitivities. If the clinical presentation allows, await sensitivities prior to commencing antibiotics to avoid contributing to antibiotic resistance. If this is not possible, empirical treatment should be started and later reviewed with the final culture results.

Ileal conduit

An ileal conduit is an incontinent diversion of urinary flow through a segment of ileum to a stoma on the abdominal wall.

The ureters are divided from the bladder and anastomosed onto a segment of ileum, usually in an end-to-end fashion. The other end of the ileal segment is brought out onto the anterior abdominal wall and spouted like any other ileostomy (**Figures 6.11, 6.12**). This is also sometimes known as a urostomy; in rare occasions these can also be made with colon. An

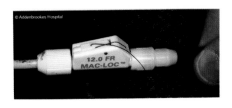

Figure 6.10 The mechanism of a typical nephrostomy tube. Before a nephrostomy is removed, the central, white plastic clip is flicked up to release the pig-tail curl on the nephrostomy.

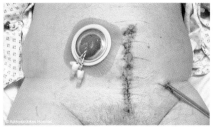

Figure 6.11 The abdomen of a man 5 days post-cystectomy demonstrating a healthy, slightly oedematous ileal conduit in the right iliac fossa. Ureteric stents are seen protruding through the stoma; these are left until fluoroscopy has demonstrated successful wound healing between each ureter and the ileal conduit. A drain is also seen in the left iliac fossa.

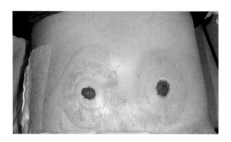

Figure 6.12 The abdomen of a female, following extensive pelvic surgery. A spouted ileal conduit is seen on the right of the patient's abdomen. An end-colostomy lies flush to the skin, to the left of the previous laparotomy incision.

Ileal conduit is most commonly performed after cystectomy, but can be used for benign disease (i.e. bladder pain syndrome or intractable incontinence). Urine is collected into a stoma bag, with or without tubing attached to it.

Problems
- Upper UTI (pyelonephritis).
- Loin pain, reduced urinary output and renal impairment due to ureteric obstruction. Causes include stenosis of the ureteroileal anastomosis or ureteric stricture.
- Parastomal hernia causing bowel obstruction.
- Symptomatic metabolic acidosis (from the use of bowel in the urinary tract) – uncommon.
- Stenosis of the bowel segment itself, causing obstruction to urinary flow.

History
- When was the operation performed and what was the indication?
- Has there been a change in urostomy output, i.e. volume, colour, smell?

- Does the patient have any pain (loin pain may indicate infection or possible renal obstruction)?
- Does the patient have fever or systemic upset?
- Have they noticed any changes with the stoma (new swelling or mass around it – which could be a hernia or collection)?

Examination
- Abdominal exam – assess for general abdominal distension or pain.
- The stoma is usually sited in the right lower quadrant. Check the stoma is healthy (should be pink); assess the surrounding skin.
- The collection bag applied around the stoma should contain urine. You will need to remove this to assess the stoma.

Investigation
- Bloods, including inflammatory markers and metabolic profile (arterial blood gas, ABG).
- Urine dip and culture: as urine has been in contact with bowel, the conduit specimen is usually positive on dipstick, so ensure a sample is sent for culture if there is a suspicion of infection.
- USS KUB to check the upper tracts if suspected of not draining; note, patients with ileal conduits may have a mild hydronephrosis presence chronically. The key is to compare the emergency imaging to previous scans to see if this is a new problem or if there has been deterioration of the hydronephrosis.
- Further investigation: other imaging that helps to look for problems with the conduit include a CT urogram, and

loopograms of the conduit. In general, these tests would be organised by urology colleagues after discussing with the radiology team.

Management
- Treat a UTI if symptomatic, ideally based on culture sensitivities.
- Monitor the urostomy output.
- Referral to urology to assess the patient.
- Ureteric obstruction will require further imaging to establish the level of obstruction and cause. Treatment is with nephrostomy insertion or insertion of special ureteric stents with a single pigtail curl in the kidney and a long straight end that exits via the conduit.
- Parastomal hernia complications require general surgery (colorectal) advice and input.
- If the patient is symptomatic from (hyperchloraemic) metabolic acidosis, treatment with sodium bicarbonate is indicated.
- Obstruction in the bowel segment of the ileal conduit can be treated with catheterisation of the stoma to help urine drain, but ultimately may require corrective surgery.

Bladder substitute/neobladder
A bladder substitute/neobladder is a continent urinary diversion made from bowel after the bladder has been removed (cystectomy).

A long segment of bowel, commonly ileum, is harvested, opened into a flat patch and then reconstructed into a sphere-shaped reservoir that will act as a bladder substitute. The ureters are reimplanted into the new bladder. The neobladder can be connected to the native urethra (orthotopic neobladder). Where this is not possible, a heterotopic neobladder is created that can be drained through an alternative route called a Mitrofanoff stoma, which is a continent, catheterisable channel (see below). The channel can be made using appendix or reconstructed ileum. It has a small open stoma on the anterior abdominal wall, and the other end is inserted into the bladder substitute. The type of neobladder chosen will depend on whether it is safe to leave the urethra *in situ* (if there is a low risk of cancer affecting the urethra), hand dexterity (ability to self-catheterise), age (higher risk of incontinence with an orthotopic bladder in older patients) and the patient's preference. The orthotopic neobladder has the advantage that, over time, the patient can urinate as they did before the procedure. After formation, voiding may have to be by timed intervals; nocturnal incontinence can be common and CISC can be necessary to complete bladder emptying.

Problems
- Urinary retention.
- Difficulty in catheterising the urethra or Mitrofanoff channel.
- UTI.
- Upper tract obstruction.
- Symptomatic metabolic acidosis.

History
- When was the operation performed and what was the indication?
- Has there been a change in urine output, i.e. volume, colour, smell?
- Does the patient have any fever, bladder pain, loin pain?

Examination
- Except from an abdominal scar, examination of the abdomen will likely be unremarkable.
- A bladder scanner may be able to assess for urinary retention.

Investigation
- Bloods, including inflammatory markers and metabolic profile (ABG).
- Urine dipstick and culture: again, urine dipstick will be positive because of the presence of urine in contact with bowel – so send urine for culture.
- Bladder scan.
- USS KUB to check the upper tracts if there is a suspicion of inadequate drainage, and assess the neobladder for post-void residuals and for bladder stones. Further investigation with CT as indicated.

Management
- Treat a UTI if symptomatic, ideally based on culture sensitivities.
- Monitor urine output.
- Referral to urology to assess the patient.
- If patients are in retention they require an indwelling catheter (either urethrally or via the Mitrofanoff).
- If it is difficult to catheterise the Mitrofanoff channel this may require cystoscopy, guidewire insertion down the channel and Seldinger catheter insertion, or alternatively, fluoroscopy of the channel, guidewire insertion and catheter insertion in radiology. Rarely, suprapubic insertion is necessary and that should only be done under radiological guidance, preferably by an interventional radiologist.
- Upper tract obstruction will need ureteric stenting or nephrostomy.

- Symptomatic metabolic acidosis should be corrected (sodium bicarbonate).

Bladder augmentation (cystoplasty)

Bladder augmentation is a surgical procedure used to treat refractory overactive bladder symptoms if conservative measures and drugs have proved ineffective. The bladder is bivalved (divided down the middle) and a flat patch of bowel (usually ileum) is anastomosed onto the top. This acts to both denervate the bladder to a degree, and enlarge the capacity of the bladder. It is also known as a clam ileocystoplasty or enterocystoplasty. Complications include incomplete bladder emptying, recurrent UTIs, mucus production, metabolic and nutritional problems and malignancy.

Problems
- UTI: cystitis and or pyelonephritis.
- Urinary retention or catheter problems.
- Haematuria: low risk of malignancy, particularly after 10 years and if the patient is self-catheterising.
- Symptomatic metabolic acidosis (uncommon).

History
- When was the procedure done? The risk of cancer is higher 10 years after the operation, and most would offer annual cystoscopy surveillance to patients at this time.
- Are recurrent UTIs a problem?
- Do they empty their bladder completely? Are they using CISC to do so?
- Have they had previous bladder calculi? How were they dealt with?

- When was the last time they had a cystoscopy?

Examination
- An abdominal scar will be apparent – either a midline laparotomy or Pfannenstiel.
- Any suprapubic tenderness?
- Any systemic signs of sepsis?

Investigation
- Bloods, including inflammatory markers and metabolic profile (ABG).
- Urine dipstick and culture.
- Bladder scan.
- USS KUB/CT KUB to look for stone formation and assess upper tracts.

Management
- Treat a UTI if symptomatic, ideally based on culture sensitivities.
- Arrange for instruction in intermittent self-catheterisation if not done previously, if there are concerns over bladder emptying.

- Organise a cystoscopy if a stone is suspected, or there is haematuria or other 'red flag' symptoms.
- Treat any metabolic abnormality if the patient is symptomatic.

Continent catheterisable channels (Mitrofanoff and Monti)

This surgical procedure creates a continent (no external collection bag) catheterisable urinary stoma between the bladder (or neobladder reservoir) and skin of the abdominal wall or umbilicus, to make an alternative route to drain the bladder. It is required in patients who have a problem with the urethra, which makes urethral catheterisation impossible or difficult to tolerate. The appendix is used most often to make the channel (Mitrofanoff) (**Figure 6.13**), or a small segment of reconstructed ileum (Monti).

Problems
- UTI.
- Obstruction to the channel (skin

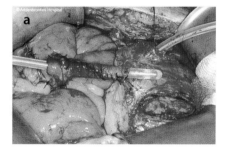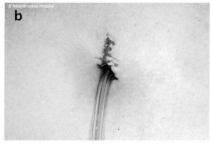

Figure 6.13 (**a**) Intra-operative image demonstrating a Mitrofanoff, a catheterisable stoma formation. Here, the appendix has been separated from the caecum and the caecum closed (left of image). The appendix has been catheterised. A suprapubic catheter is seen in the native bladder (right of image); (**b**) the umbilical area following surgery. A temporary silicone catheter is left within the appendix to allow healing.

stenosis or stenosis within the channel or where it inserts into the bladder).
- Leaking or bypassing.

Management
- Infection: the risk is reduced by drinking plenty of fluids and ensuring complete emptying of the bladder and good catheterisation technique.
- Stenosis: if it becomes difficult for the individual to pass their usual catheter they will need to seek urgent medical attention. In the first instance the catheter can be left indwelling and then reassessed if surgical revision is indicated. The patient will invariably be the expert at catheterising their own stoma. If they are unable to pass a catheter, it is not unreasonable for a urologist to try to catheterise but fluoroscopy-guided insertion may well become necessary. Occasionally the patient will require a formal channel dilatation in theatre.
- Leaking: either due to a high bladder pressure or a problem with the insertion of the channel into the bladder (weakness of the antirefluxing mechanism).

Artificial urinary sphincters

An artificial urinary sphincter (AUS) is a surgical device used to treat stress incontinence related to sphincter deficiency in men and women. It is a closed system comprising an inflatable cuff placed at the bulbar urethra in men or bladder neck, a pressure-regulating reservoir balloon located in the abdomen (extraperitoneal) and an activating pump sited in the scrotum or labia majora (**Figures 6.14 and 6.15**).

When the pump is squeezed, fluid in

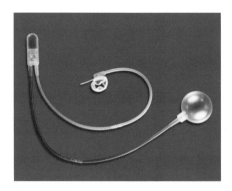

Figure 6.14 The internal mechanism of an AUS device (AMS 800). Water is transferred from the inflatable cuff to the pressure-regulating balloon reservoir by multiple squeezes of the control pump, which allows voiding. (Image courtesy of Boston Scientific.)

the cuff is transferred to the reservoir so that the pressure exerted on the urethra is reduced (cuff deactivated), allowing voiding to occur, after which the cuff automatically refills over the subsequent few minutes.

Problems
- Infection of the device: may manifest as the AUS not working (urinary incontinence or potentially urinary retention), skin infection over the components, erosion of a component through the skin.
- Urinary retention with the AUS working (i.e. due to other causes).

Management
- Treat infection aggressively with antibiotics. An infected device often culminates in the need to explant/remove the AUS, wait 6 months and then reinsert another device.

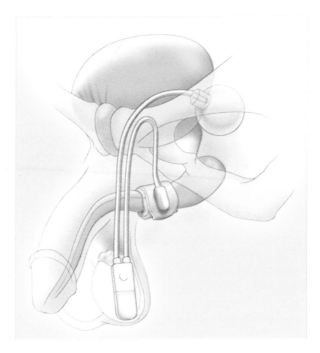

Figure 6.15 Diagram demonstrating the usual positioning of a male AUS device. The balloon reservoir is placed in the lower abdomen, the cuff surrounds the urethra (or bladder neck) circumferentially, with the pump palpable in the scrotum. (Image courtesy of Boston Scientific.)

- NEVER catheterise a patient with an AUS unless the device has been deactivated – call a urologist. Inadvertent catheterisation with the urethral cuff inflated can result in cuff erosion and urethral injury, requiring urethral repair and removal of the device.
- If a urethral catheter is required, a urologist will deactivate the sphincter and then pass the smallest possible catheter (12 Fr). An alternative would be suprapubic catheter insertion, taking care to stay away from where the balloon reservoir is implanted in the abdomen.

- Mild hydronephrosis is commonly present with a ureteric stent *in situ* and should not be a cause for concern unless the patient is unwell.

- If a patient presents with a nephrostomy problem, establish whether the tube is still draining, and if not, flush it gently to unblock it. If flushing does not resolve the situation, consider imaging to assess whether the tube is displaced and requires reinsertion.

- Never remove a nephrostomy without first releasing the locking thread – some nephrostomies should be removed under fluoroscopic guidance.

- In the context of problems with ileal conduits, imaging of the upper tracts can identify if there is a new, or change to an existing, hydronephrosis indicating possible upper urinary tract obstruction. Always compare the anatomy to old scans to identify if this is a new or pre-existing finding.

- Patients with a previous cystoplasty who report haematuria require urgent cystoscopic investigation, due to increased risks of neoplasia.

- Problems with catheterising continent catheterisable channels are relatively common and require specialist urological input.

- Catheterisation of patients with artificial urinary sphincters should only be performed by those with knowledge of how to deactivate the device.

References

1   The National Institute for Health and Care Excellence (NICE). Diagnosis and management of adults at risk of and with metastatic spinal cord compression. NICE guidelines (CG75), November 2008.

Chapter 7

Procedures in Urology

Adam Nelson and Suzanne Biers[1,2,3] / Michal Sut[4]

URETHRAL CATHETERISATION[1]

Urethral catheterisation of the urinary bladder is a core skill not just for the urologist, but for all medical practitioners. The principal indications and relative contraindications for urethral catheter–isation are shown in *Box 7.1*. Note also the situations where advice should be sought from a urology consultant before attempting catheterisation.

Types of catheter

For the purposes of this chapter, all catheters described will be variations of the Foley catheter, which has an inflatable balloon at the tip to keep the catheter in place. A typical catheter is also known as a '2-way catheter' as it has two lumens. One lumen drains urine from the bladder and a much smaller second channel is used to fill or empty the balloon. Three-way catheters have an additional channel that may be used for irrigation. Catheters are typically made from either coated latex or silicone (**Figure 7.1**). Latex catheters tend to be for short-term use (less than 4 weeks), whereas silicone catheters may be left in place for up to 12 weeks. Silicone catheters are stiffer, which may make them easier to

Box 7.1 Indications for urethral catheterisation.

- Urinary retention (acute and chronic).
- Monitoring of urine output.
- Post-operative decompression of the bladder (e.g. following bladder repair).
- Bladder washout/irrigation for visible haematuria.

Consider referral to urology

- Recent/post-operative radical prostatectomy.
- Pelvic trauma with haematuria/blood at meatus (a single attempt by an experienced doctor is acceptable).
- Known urethral stricture disease.
- Artificial urinary sphincter *in situ*.

insert in certain patients (e.g. where there is resistance from an enlarged prostate) and as a result are often used if attempts at insertion of a latex catheter have failed. In patients with a latex allergy, silicone catheters can be used safely.

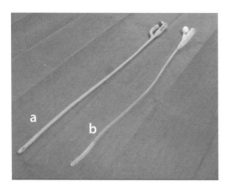

Figure 7.1 Examples of 2-way Foley catheters in coated latex (**a**) and silicone (**b**).

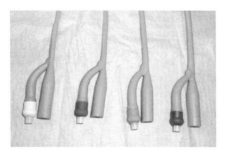

Figure 7.2 2-way Foley catheters demonstrating the colours associated with common sizes. White=12 Fr, green=14 Fr, orange=16 Fr, red=18 Fr.

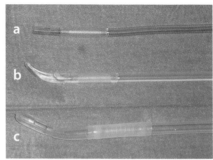

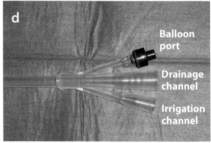

Figure 7.3 Examples of specialist catheters. (**a**) Council tip catheter; (**b**) Tiemann tip catheter; (**c**) coudé tip 3-way catheter; (**d**) components of a 3-way catheter.

Catheters are sized according to their external diameter. The diameter is reported in 'French' (Fr), which equates to 1/3 of a millimetre. Therefore, an 18 Fr catheter has a diameter of 6mm. The unit 'Charrière' (Ch) is used interchangeably with 'French', after the scale's inventor. A colour coding system is used that permits easy identification of catheter size (**Figure 7.2**). As a general rule, the smallest calibre catheter that is fit for purpose should be used to minimise the risk of urethral trauma. Male length catheters are 40–45cm in length. Shorter female catheters are rarely available because of the risks associated with selecting too short a catheter for male catheterisation.

Specialist catheters
A number of catheters are made with specific features to make them useful in particular contexts (**Figure 7.3**):

• Tiemann tip: a curved, narrow-tipped catheter usually made from silicone. A useful catheter for men with enlarged prostates where the curved tip helps pass the U-bend of the bulbar urethra, or women with a difficult to find urethral meatus high on the anterior vaginal wall.

- Straight/Couvelaire tip 3-way: a large-bore catheter with an additional lumen to allow instillation of fluid into the bladder and a wide opening to allow passage of debris or blood clots. These are 18–24 Fr calibre and used for bladder irrigation or washout in the event of visible haematuria with clot retention. Larger-calibre catheters will accept a larger volume of fluid in the balloon and the capacity is documented on the catheter or packaging.
- Coudé tip: a wide-bore, curved-tip catheter (coudé is French for elbow). Typically found on large (18–24 Fr) 3-way catheters as described above. Used for bladder irrigation/washout following transurethral prostatectomy as the curved tip enables smooth passage across the 'U-bend' of the bulbar urethra and resected prostate bed.
- Council tip: a straight, silicone catheter with an open, end-on hole in the tip. This catheter can be passed over a guidewire, and is therefore typically used in flexible cystoscopy-guided urethral catheterisation. Subsequently, it is possible to exchange catheters over a guidewire, without the need for further cystoscopy.

Technique of urethral catheterisation

As with any medical procedure, training in catheterisation should only be undertaken under the supervision of a competent person. The description below should, however, serve as initial preparation for those learning the procedure, or as an aide-mémoire for those who have been previously trained:

- Establish a clear indication for urethral catheterisation, and identify situations where urology input should be sought.
- Explain to the patient the nature of the procedure, the possible complications (see later section) and seek consent from the patient.
- Consider antibiotic prophylaxis, particularly if there have been multiple attempts at catheterisation, a history of recurrent urinary tract infection (UTI) or recent instrumentation of the urinary tract.
- Ensure all necessary equipment is within easy reach (*Box 7.2*).
- Wash hands and maintain a sterile technique throughout.

Box 7.2 Basic equipment.

- Sterile dressing pack.
- Sterile saline to clean glans/vulva.
- Sterile gloves.
- Local anaesthetic lubricant jelly.
- Catheter (selected according to indication).
- Syringe with sterile water (not saline) for catheter balloon (usually 10ml syringe).
- Catheter bag.

In men:
- Ensure you have selected a male length catheter. A female length catheter will not reach the male bladder and will cause significant trauma if the balloon is inflated within the urethra.
- Retract the foreskin if present and clean the glans with sterile saline.
- With the patient supine, grasp the penis with a swab and raise it vertically.
- Gently insert local anaesthetic lubricant jelly into the urethral meatus. Spill some jelly on the glans around the meatus, as this will lubricate the catheter as it passes.
- With the penis pointing upwards, insert the catheter. When you feel the catheter is in the bulbar urethra, angle the penis to the patient's feet. Insert the catheter 'to the hilt,' ensuring that it does not spring back when released. A catheter that springs back may have coiled in the bulbar or prostatic urethra.
- Wait for drainage of urine to confirm correct placement within the bladder. If not certain, try aspirating through the catheter lumen as lubricant jelly may inhibit the flow.
- Inflate the balloon slowly with sterile water. Most 2-way catheter balloons have a 10ml balloon. Watch the patient's face while doing so; if he experiences any pain, deflate the balloon immediately.
- Replace the foreskin, if present.
- Attach the appropriate catheter bag.

In women:
- A male or female length catheter may be used in a female patient.
- With the patient supine, ask her to bend the knees, feet together and then place the knees apart. Gently spread the labia with one hand and with the other hand, clean the vulva and urethra with saline.
- Locate the external urethral meatus, bearing in mind that it may be located on the anterior vaginal wall, particularly in post-menopausal women.
- Insert a few millilitres of local anaesthetic lubricant jelly into the meatus.
- Insert the catheter until urine drains, or until more than 5cm of the catheter has passed.
- Inflate the balloon with sterile water. Watch the patient's face while doing so; if she experiences any pain, deflate the balloon immediately.
- Attach the appropriate catheter bag.

Documentation
After urethral catheterisation, the following details should be recorded in the patient's notes:

- The indication for the catheter.
- Consent and whether a chaperone was present.
- Whether antibiotic prophylaxis was given.
- The type of catheter used, and the number of attempts required for successful insertion.
- The volume of water in the balloon.
- The volume of urine drained from the bladder immediately following catheterisation (the residual volume). This is particularly important as it will often determine the subsequent management of patients presenting with urinary retention.
- Plan for subsequent catheter removal/renewal as appropriate.

Figure 7.4 Algorithm for difficult catheterisation.

Indication: decompression of urinary tract and direct monitoring of urine output.
Rationale: minimise the risk of sepsis, trauma to the urinary tract or patient discomfort.

Step 1

Patient check
- Clear indication?
- Observations
- Verbal consent
- Analgesia
- Antibiotic prophylaxis? (Check antimicrobial prophylaxis guidelines)

DO NOT ATTEMPT CATHETERISATION for these patients:
1. Post-op radical prostatectomies
2. Mitrofanoff conduits
3. Known urethral strictures
4. Pelvic trauma with haematuria

Call UROLOGY

Equipment check
- Correct catheter type and size
- 10-30ml water + syringe for balloon
- Local anaesthetic lubricant gel
- Saline or alternative cleaning solution
- Sterile dressing pack
- Sterile gloves
- Catheter drainage bag

Step 2

Patient check
- Observations
- Offer of analgesia
- Reassess indication
- Consider antimicrobial prophylaxis if significant iatrogenic trauma

Tips and tricks!
- Ensure the patient is relaxed
- Encourage urination
- Generous use of local anaesthetic lubricant
- Increase catheter size and/or rigidity (100% silicone)
- Curved tip catheter for possible prostatic obstruction if experienced

If after 2 attempts, no success or iatrogenic trauma
CONTACT UROLOGY

Step 3 – Specialty-led

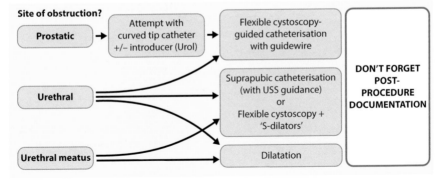

Tips and tricks

Difficult female catheterisation

Occasionally it can be difficult to identify the female external urethral meatus. Where practical, place the patient's bottom onto a pillow. This tilts the pelvis forward and can make it easier to identify the urethra. Should this fail, after careful explanation and verbal consent, insertion of a finger may occlude the lumen of the vagina and lead the catheter into the urethral meatus. It is also possible to sometimes feel the urethral meatus with the tip of the finger helping the direction of the catheter. Alternatively, place the patient in the left lateral position, lift the uppermost leg in the air, and place a Sims speculum into the posterior part of the vagina to help visualise the anterior vaginal wall and urethra.

Unable to site a catheter and no specialist help available

If the patient has a palpable bladder and you are unable to get help to place either a urethral catheter or suprapubic catheter, it is possible to aspirate the bladder suprapubically to make the patient with acute painful urinary retention comfortable until help is available. Take patient consent, and prepare the lower abdomen with iodine solution and drapes. Inject 5–10ml 1% lignocaine into the skin 2cm above the symphysis pubis in the midline, and also towards the bladder. Use a green needle and 50ml syringe. Direct the needle perpendicular to the skin and slightly downward, aspirate until you reach the bladder. A 3-way tap can be attached to the end of the needle. Urine can then be removed in small aliquots until the patient feels more comfortable.

Key Points

- Establish the indication for catheterisation and the absence of any contraindications where specialist urology input may be required.
- Select a catheter appropriate for the indication and the patient's past medical history.
- Maintain aseptic technique throughout.
- In the event of failure, follow the difficult catheterisation algorithm (**Figure 7.4**).
- Always remember to replace the foreskin in a man.
- Clearly document the procedure.
- Suprapubic aspirations can be used as a temporising measure when a patient is in retention, catheter insertion has failed and no specialist help is immediately available.

SUPRAPUBIC CATHETERISATION[2]

Suprapubic catheterisation involves the insertion of a Foley catheter through the suprapubic region of the anterior abdominal wall, directly into the urinary bladder. In the elective setting, it may be used for patients who lack the manual dexterity or cognitive ability to perform clean intermittent self-catheterisation (CISC) or as an alternative in patients otherwise reliant on a long-term indwelling urethral catheter. Elective indications for a suprapubic catheter (SPC) include chronic urinary retention due to bladder outlet obstruction or bladder underactivity, or for voiding dysfunction seen in spinal cord injury and neuropathic bladder. Postoperatively, a SPC is often used after bladder repair or reconstruction to decompress the bladder and facilitate healing and is usually combined with a urethral catheter in that setting. The advantages of SPCs over a urethral catheter for long-term use is that it avoids trauma to the soft tissues of the urethra (**Figure 7.5**), which can result in a patulous urethra and incontinence in women, and spatulation or splitting of the glans and penile shaft in men.

The focus of this chapter, however, will be on the use of SPC insertion in the emergency setting (*Box 7.3*). Guidance published by the British Association of Urological Surgeons (BAUS)[1] summarises many of the relevant issues relating to the use of SPCs (*Box 7.4*).

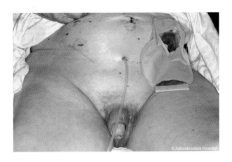

Figure 7.5 An elderly man with a recently placed suprapubic catheter. This catheter and the defunctioning colostomy were placed to help in the management of a complex colovesical fistula and penile abscess.

Box 7.3 Emergency SPC insertion.

Indications

- Acute, painful urinary retention where urethral catheterisation has failed.
- Urethral injury, e.g. pelvic trauma.

Contraindications

- Impalpable bladder.
- Known bladder cancer.
- Anticoagulated patient.
- Abdominal wall sepsis.
- Subcutaneous vascular graft in suprapubic region, e.g. femorofemoral crossover graft
- Previous abdominal/pelvic surgery (requires an open cystotomy approach).

Box 7.4 BAUS guidance on SPC insertion.[1]

- In the patient with a palpable bladder and no previous abdominal surgery, blind percutaneous SPC insertion is reasonable if urine can be easily aspirated with a needle at the planned insertion site.

- Blind insertion should not be performed in the patient with previous abdominal surgery and an impalpable bladder. Consider using ultrasound scanning (USS) or cystoscopy to assist the procedure.

- In patients with previous surgery or where distension of the bladder is not possible, an open technique of insertion should be used.

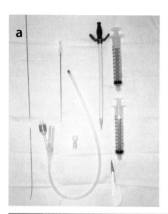

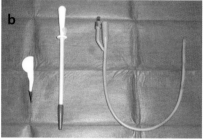

Figure 7.6 (**a**) Components of the Mediplus Ltd S-Cath™ system (images used with permission); (**b**) components of the Bard™ suprapubic catheter set.

Techniques for insertion of a percutaneous SPC

There are two commonly used methods used for emergency percutaneous insertion of a SPC (**Figure 7.6**). Firstly, a trocar-based technique (e.g. BARD® suprapubic kit) and secondly, a Seldinger-based technique (e.g. Mediplus Ltd. S-Cath™ system suprapubic Catheterisation with Seldinger technique). As with any medical procedure, training in suprapubic catheterisation should only be undertaken under the supervision of a competent person. The description below should however serve as initial preparation for those learning the procedure, or an aide-mémoire for those who have been previously trained.

Trocar-based technique

- Establish a clear indication for a SPC.
- Explain to the patient the nature of the procedure, the possible risks (*Box 7.5*) and seek consent from the patient.
- Give antibiotic prophylaxis (e.g. gentamicin 80mg IV/IM).
- Ensure all necessary equipment has been checked and is present within easy reach.
- Wash hands and maintain a sterile technique throughout.
- Identify the insertion site, 2cm above the symphysis pubis in the midline.
- Where available, obtain USS confirmation that no bowel is

interposed between the anterior abdominal wall and the bladder at the proposed insertion site.

- Prepare the lower abdomen with antiseptic solution (e.g. betadine).
- Administer local anaesthesia along the planned track, until urine is aspirated from the bladder (10ml 1% lignocaine, remembering to aspirate first to ensure you are not injecting into a blood vessel).
- Make a small, stab skin incision at the insertion site with a blade. It is very important to cut down with the blade onto the rectus sheath to incise it. Cutting the rectus sheath feels like scraping the grit with the blade, which limits the depth of the incision.
- Insert the SPC introducer (trocar with a sheath) at an angle perpendicular to the bladder wall (a gentle twisting motion may be required). Apply gentle and controlled pressure in this direction. If the incision of the rectus sheath was done appropriately then a little resistance on entering the bladder is expected. There is often a slight give at this point, and you will see urine draining out of the sheath, which confirms your placement in the bladder.
- Quickly (before the bladder empties) remove the trocar, leaving the outer sheath in place and insert the Foley catheter down the channel of the sheath.
- Inflate the catheter balloon with 10ml water.
- Divide and remove the sheath (this then peels off).
- Attach an appropriate catheter drainage bag. In the emergency setting, you may be expecting large urinary residual or post-obstructive diuresis, so a urometer bag may be best to start with.

Seldinger-based technique

- Establish a clear indication for a SPC.
- Explain to the patient the nature of the procedure, the possible risks (*Box 7.5*) and seek consent from the patient.
- Give antibiotic prophylaxis (e.g. gentamicin 80mg IV/IM).
- Ensure all necessary equipment has been checked and is present within reach.
- Wash hands and maintain a sterile technique throughout.
- Identify the insertion site, 2cm above the symphysis pubis in the midline.
- Where available, obtain USS confirmation that no bowel is

Box 7.5 Risks of SPC insertion.[2]

- Common (>10%): haematuria.
- Occasional (2–10%):
  › UTI.
  › Recurrent catheter blockages.
  › Bladder discomfort.
  › Persistent urethral leakage of urine.
  › Development of stones/debris in the bladder, which may require surgical treatment.
- Rare (<2%):
  › Heavy bleeding requiring bladder irrigation or evacuation of clot.
  › Injury to bowel or other abdominal organs.
  › Hospital-acquired infection (e.g. methicillin-resistant *Staphylococcus aureus*, *Clostridium difficile*).

interposed between the anterior abdominal wall and the bladder at the proposed insertion site.

- Prepare the lower abdomen with antiseptic solution.
- Using the syringe and long fine needle included in the set, administer local anaesthesia along the planned track, until urine is aspirated from the bladder (**Figure 7.7**: Step 1).
- Remove the syringe from the needle, maintaining the needle in position within the bladder (**Figure 7.7**: Step 2).
- Pass the guidewire down the needle into the bladder, then remove the

needle leaving the guidewire in place (**Figure 7.7**: Step 3).

- Make a small, stab incision adjacent to the guidewire into the puncture site. Then advance the blade along the wire toward the rectus muscle. As with the previous technique it is important to cut down to the rectus sheath and incise it (which would feel like scraping the grit with the blade).
- Insert the trocar over the guidewire into the bladder (**Figure 7.7**: Step 4).
- Remove the guidewire and trocar, leaving the outer sheath in place (**Figure 7.7**: Step 5).

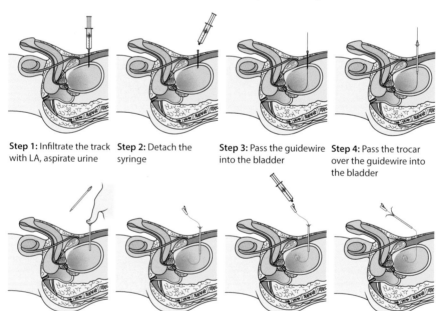

Step 1: Infiltrate the track with LA, aspirate urine

Step 2: Detach the syringe

Step 3: Pass the guidewire into the bladder

Step 4: Pass the trocar over the guidewire into the bladder

Step 5: Remove the guidewire and inner trocar leaving the outer sheath in the bladder

Step 6: Pass the Foley catheter down the sheath into the bladder

Step 7: Inflate the catheter balloon

Step 8: Split and remove the outer sheath

Figure 7.7 Insertion of Mediplus Ltd. S-Cath™ System. Suprapubic catheterisation with the Seldinger technique. (Images used with permission.)

- Quickly pass the Foley catheter down the outer sheath and inflate the catheter balloon with 10ml water before the bladder empties (**Figure 7.7**: Steps 6, 7).
- Divide and remove the sheath (**Figure 7.7**: Step 8).
- Attach an appropriate catheter drainage bag.

Replacement/exchange of an existing suprapubic catheter

- Assemble the kit required as for urethral catheterisation. Use the same catheter size and type that you are to remove.
- Place a sterile drape on the area and clean.
- Deflate the balloon and remove the existing catheter.
- Immediately insert lubricant gel into the tract, and advance a new catheter.
- After return of urine, advance the catheter slightly further, to avoid inflating the balloon in the urinary SPC tract.
- Inflate the balloon carefully, observing the patient's face for any discomfort. There is a small risk of the catheter migrating into the urethra, especially in females. Visually check the female urethra.

- Ensure the catheter is freely mobile in the tract and withdraw the catheter so that the balloon is in contact with the anterior bladder wall.
- Attach a drainage bag, securing tubing to avoid trauma.

Documentation

After suprapubic catheterisation, the following details should be recorded in the patient's notes:

- The indication for the SPC.
- Consent.
- Antibiotic prophylaxis given.
- USS confirmation of site, where available.
- Local anaesthesia administered.
- The technique used and number of attempts required for successful insertion.
- The volume of water in the balloon.
- The volume of urine drained from the bladder immediately following catheterisation (the residual volume). This is particularly important, as it will often determine the subsequent management of patients presenting with urinary retention.

Key Points

- BAUS has published helpful guidance on SPC insertion.
- Trocar-based and Seldinger-based techniques are both established.
- Patients must be clearly informed of the potential risks of the procedure in order to give informed consent.
- Beware of the contraindications to suprapubic catheter insertion.
- Clear documentation of the indication, the procedure and the volume/colour of the urine and volume of urine drained after the procedure is essential.

CATHETER COMPLICATIONS[3]

Catheter complications are common, and referrals relating to catheter-associated issues have been shown to make up around 30% of the on-call workload of a large, tertiary-referral urology department[3]. In this chapter we review some of the common catheter-related complications with simple steps to help manage them and to inform onward referrals if necessary.

Complications of urethral catheter insertion

False passage

Attempts at male catheterisation can result in urethral trauma, where a 'false passage' is formed by the catheter penetrating the urethra and entering the surrounding tissues. This typically occurs in the 'U-bend' of the bulbar urethra. It is recognised by an inability to pass a catheter beyond the prostate, urethral bleeding and often pain. False passages can also occur when attempting to pass a catheter in a patient with a urethral stricture. False passage formation can often be avoided by good catheterisation technique.

Management
- Stop further attempts at catheter insertion.
- Consider administration of a stat dose of a broad-spectrum antibiotic such as co-amoxiclav or gentamicin.
- Contact the urology team for assistance as cystoscopically-guided insertion of a urethral catheter or SPC may be required.

Balloon inflated in the prostatic urethra

If the male catheter isn't fully advanced into

the bladder, the tip of the catheter may still be in the prostatic urethra. Inflation of the balloon causes trauma, pain and bleeding (or persistent haematuria). Urine may or may not be draining from the catheter depending on the precise location of the catheter tip. It may be noted that the length of catheter protruding from the end of the penis is longer than usual.

Management
- Deflate the catheter balloon immediately.
- Consider administration of a stat dose of a broad-spectrum antibiotic such as co-amoxiclav or gentamicin.
- Gently attempt to fully advance the catheter into the bladder.
- Do not inflate the balloon until urine is seen to drain from the catheter.
- Seek urology help if unsuccessful or if there is heavy bleeding.

Difficult female catheterisation

Occasionally it can be difficult to visualise the female external urethral meatus for catheterisation. This is more common in post-menopausal women where the meatus can retract up the anterior vaginal wall. Consider the stepwise approach detailed below.

Management
- With the patient in the lithotomy position, place a pillow underneath her pelvis to lift it and rotate the meatus into view.
- Place a gloved and lubricated index finger onto the anterior vaginal wall to palpate the meatus. Keeping the fingertip on the meatus, pass a catheter down the palmar surface of your finger and direct it into the urethra. Consider

using a Tiemann tip catheter, as the angulated tip will help.

- Alternatively, place the patient in the left lateral position with the knees bent to the chest. Use a Sims speculum to retract the posterior vaginal wall, allowing visualisation of the anterior vaginal wall and urethral meatus (**Figure 7.8**).
- If all of the above are unsuccessful, contact urology for consideration of cystoscopically-guided catheter or SPC insertion.

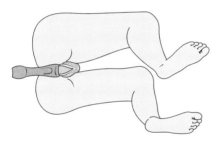

Figure 7.8 A Sims speculum can be useful to retract the posterior vaginal wall to allow visualisation of the anterior vaginal wall and urethral meatus.

Tight phimosis/non-retractile foreskin

In adult men, phimosis (physiological or secondary to balanitis xerotica obliterans) can cause difficulty with urethral catheterisation. It may be so severe that the preputial opening appears to be only 'pinhole'-sized

Management

- Attempt gentle retraction or movement of the foreskin to try and visualise the urethral meatus. If the meatus can be visualised, sterilise the exposed glans along with the rest of the procedural field as normal and proceed in the usual manner.
- If attempted retraction does not permit visualisation, try pulling the foreskin upwards instead. This will often reveal an opening and access to the glans. Gently insert the tip of a syringe, which can then be used to 'wash out' under the foreskin with antiseptic solution to clean the field. The tip of the syringe of lubricating gel can then be guided blindly with the aid of careful palpation into the urethral meatus. In a similar fashion, the tip of the lubricated catheter can then be guided blindly with palpation into the urethral opening and subsequently to the bladder. Proceed gently, and ensure that urine drains before inflating the catheter balloon.
- If these are not successful, then a urologist should be contacted for assistance. This will usually entail placement of a local anaesthetic penile block, followed by forceps dilatation of the preputial opening to visualise the meatus. Occasionally a dorsal slit may be required, or alternative ways to drain the bladder can be considered such as insertion of a suprapubic catheter.

Paraphimosis

When catheterising uncircumcised male patients, it is essential to replace the retracted foreskin at the end of the procedure. Failure to do so can lead to paraphimosis, where the preputial opening forms a tight band around the base of the glans (see page 81). This leads to venous congestion and swelling of the inner preputial layer. If left untreated, this can result in massive swelling and eventual ischaemic necrosis of the glans penis. Also, refer to page 82 for management.

Management
- If competent to do so, administer a regional anaesthetic penile block. Wait to ensure a good block is achieved (see pages 166–170).
- Coat the glans and prepuce in lidocaine jelly (e.g. Instillagel®).
- With the penis wrapped in gauze, squeeze the oedematous inner prepuce firmly, and hold for 10 minutes (hence the need for good anaesthesia). The aim is to squeeze the fluid out of the oedematous tissue.
- With the index and middle fingers of each hand hooked under the phimotic band and the thumbs on the tip of the glans, pull the phimotic band over the head of the glans to reduce the paraphimosis. Ensure the phimotic band actually comes over the glans and not just the inner prepuce.

Buried penis/genitoscrotal oedema
Overweight men and men with large inguinoscrotal hernias may present with some difficulty with catheterisation due to a 'buried penis'. This may be due to a large fat pad over the pubic symphysis or the presence of a hernial swelling. Genitoscrotal oedema typically occurs in patients in intensive care who have been bed-bound for some time with sepsis, congestive heart disease or multi-organ failure and typically low serum albumin.

Management
- If a hernia is present, attempt gentle reduction of the hernia to reveal the penis.
- If a large fat pad is present, press the fingers in towards the base of the penis to help it protrude.
- If oedema is present, gently squeeze the oedema out of the penile skin, which will allow retraction and a better grasp of the penile shaft for catheterisation to proceed.
- Occasionally an assistant is required to retract or control the obstructing tissues.

Decompression haematuria
This occurs after relieving high-pressure chronic urinary retention in up to 16% of cases[4]. It is thought to occur as a result of micro-injury to the capillaries of the urothelium lining the bladder. The bleeding is typically light (rosé wine-coloured) and is self-limiting. In the event of dark haematuria (red wine-coloured) with passage of clots, then the following management is necessary.

Management
- Insert a large-bore (18–22 Fr) 3-way urethral catheter.
- Perform a gentle bladder washout with 50ml instillation/aspiration of sterile saline.
- Contact urology for advice regarding formal bladder irrigation.
- Carefully monitor urine output and renal function for post-obstructive diuresis.

Hypospadias
In hypospadias, the external urethral meatus lies somewhere along the ventral aspect of the penis between the glans and perineum, proximal to the normal anatomical position. Catheterisation can usually be performed as normal; however, it is worth noting that there may be a degree of meatal stenosis.

If the catheter tip does not pass easily, contact urology for assistance. They may perform meatal dilatation.

Meatal stenosis

In meatal stenosis the external urethral opening of the glans penis is too tight to allow catheterisation. This should be referred to a urologist for meatal dilatation under local anaesthesia. False passage formation is a significant risk, and so the inexperienced clinician should not attempt this procedure. If dilatation is unsuccessful, or urethral trauma is caused, then SPC placement is typically required.

Catheter inserted into a ureter

This is a very rare complication of catheter insertion, but potentially devastating if unrecognised. It has been described in patients with spinal cord injury and is thought to arise as a result of a small, incompetent bladder with vesicoureteric reflux leading to dilation of the ureteric orifices[5]. Inflation of the catheter balloon leads to abdominal/loin pain and haematuria, with immediate relief of pain on deflation of the balloon.

Management

- In patients with spinal cord injury, be aware of the external length of the catheter once positioned (i.e. the tubing would be very short in this case).
- If ureteric injury is suspected, perform urgent computed tomography (CT) urography to establish the nature of the injury.
- Administer a broad-spectrum antibiotic such as co-amoxiclav or gentamicin.
- Refer to urology.

Allergic reaction

This complication is rare. However, many urinary catheters are still composed of latex, which is a common allergen. Always check allergy status before starting catheterisation. If you suspect an allergic reaction, or anaphylaxis, remove the precipitant (the catheter) and manage anaphylaxis according to the Resuscitation Council guidelines. Minor reactions might settle with removal of the trigger and antihistamines. Ensure that the patient is aware of the allergy and it is clearly documented in their patient record and refer for allergy testing.

Complications of catheters *in situ*

Bladder spasms/urinary bypassing/catheter expulsion

With a catheter *in situ*, patients may complain of intermittent suprapubic discomfort and a sudden feeling of urgency to void. This may be accompanied by leakage of urine around the outside of the catheter (bypassing) or in female patients expulsion of the catheter with the balloon inflated. These three are all caused by bladder spasm, an overactive bladder contraction in response to the irritative presence of the catheter in the bladder.

Management

- Exclude blockage of the catheter as a potential cause. Consider a gentle bladder washout if debris is apparent in the catheter, as this may be causing intermittent blockages. Replace the catheter if it is obviously blocked.
- Consider prescribing an anticholinergic medication such as oxybutynin (if not contraindicated).

- Single expulsion of a catheter with the balloon inflated is unlikely to cause significant trauma. If it happens repeatedly, refer to urology for advice. Avoid using a larger catheter or inflating the balloon with more fluid, as this can exacerbate urethral injury if the catheter is expelled again.

Blood/debris in the catheter tubing and bag

This is very common, particularly with long-term catheters *in situ*. Heavy bleeding (red wine-coloured urine) or blood clots can lead to catheter blockages (clot retention), and requires urgent treatment (see management below). Lighter haematuria also requires investigation, treatment of any reversible causes (raised International Normalised Ratio [INR], UTI) and later investigation (as appropriate) to exclude a tumour or stones.

Management

- If significant haematuria or large blood clots are present, remove the original catheter and insert a larger-calibre (18–22 Fr) 3-way catheter.
- Perform a gentle bladder washout as above.
- Refer to urology for advice regarding formal bladder irrigation if haematuria continues.
- Identify and treat the underlying cause of the haematuria (see pages 52–58).

Blockages

For other types of catheter blockage ensure there are no kinks or twists in the catheter tubing, and that the catheter bag is below the level of the bladder. If still not draining, palpate the lower abdomen or perform a bladder scan to establish if the bladder is full or if the patient is in fact anuric or oliguric as the cause of their 'poor catheter drainage'. If the bladder is full and the catheter is still blocked, attempt a gentle flush of the catheter with 30ml sterile saline. If unsuccessful, replace the catheter.

Encrustation and stone formation

Long-term urethral and SPCs are both associated with an increased risk of bladder stone formation, particularly in spinal cord-injured patients. It has been shown that approximately 25% of patients with long-term catheters will develop bladder stones, with a 4% annual risk of stone formation[6]. Bladder stones may cause bladder spasm, catheter bypassing and recurrent catheter blockages. Visible encrustation of the catheter when removed is associated with bladder stone formation and should prompt assessment for the presence of a bladder stone[7].

Management

- If bladder stones are suspected, a plain abdominal X-ray should be performed.
- Treat bladder spasm if present as above and any symptomatic UTI.
- If stones are found, refer to urology for further management.
- Most bladder stones will require endoscopic removal under general anaesthetic (cystolitholapaxy with laser fragmentation of the stone).
- Counsel patients to increase fluid intake (to avoid UTI and further encrustation and stone formation around the catheter). The addition of fresh lemon juice to drinking water can reduce the risk of catheter encrustation as it contains citric acid.

Catheter-associated UTI (CAUTI)

Indwelling catheters increase the risk of UTI. Bacteria may gain entry into the bladder during insertion of the catheter or subsequent manipulation of the catheter or drainage system. Catheters promote bacterial colonisation by providing a surface for adhesion and they cause urothelial irritation. In catheterised patients, the daily incidence of bacteriuria is 3–10%. Between 10% and 30% of patients who undergo short-term catheterisation (up to 4 days) develop asymptomatic bacteriuria. Between 90% and 100% of patients who undergo long-term catheterisation develop bacteriuria. About 80% of hospital-acquired UTIs are related to urethral catheterisation.

Management

- CAUTI only needs to be treated if symptomatic (fever, cystitis/pain, new confusion).
- If a catheter has been *in situ* for more than 7 days, change to a new catheter when starting antibiotics for CAUTI.
- Minimise handling of the catheter and maximise use of closed-loop drainage systems to reduce the risk of further CAUTI.
- Document the indication for the catheter and an anticipated removal date (if not long-term), and remove the catheter as soon as it is no longer needed.

Soft tissue erosion/penile spatulation

Also known as acquired, iatrogenic or traumatic hypospadias, this is a complication of long-term urethral male catheterisation. It occurs as a result of continual downward pressure from the catheter on the ventral surface of the urethra. Whilst it looks very alarming (**Figure 7.9**), it is usually painless and it is a chronic condition that does not require urgent urological review. Concerned patients should be seen in the outpatient clinic to discuss alternative forms of bladder drainage such as SPC insertion or intermittent catheterisation (+/- surgical repair of hypospadias). Erosion can be minimised by using the softest catheter available and using a catheter strap or restrainer (usually attached to the upper thigh).

Psychological impact

Catheters can carry a significant psychological burden, affecting an individual's self-image and sexual function amongst other impacts. Catheters should only be used when indicated, and measures to maximise independence and normality should be sought; for instance, using

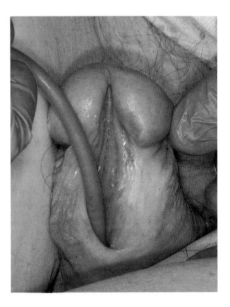

Figure 7.9 Iatrogenic hypospadias as a consequence of long-term male urethral catheterisation.

flip-flow valves as opposed to leg bags, if appropriate, which will allow the patient to go swimming and move more freely.

Complications of urethral catheter removal

Unable to deflate balloon and remove catheter

Occasionally, the retaining balloon of the Foley catheter cannot be deflated. This may occur as a result of failure of the valve mechanism, blockage of the inflation channel, or rarely, formation of salt crystals as a result of the balloon having been filled with normal saline instead of water[8]. The following are suggested as a step-wise approach to resolving this problem. The urology team should be involved if needing to progress beyond the first 3 steps described below.

Management
- First try to aspirate more fluid from the balloon, as occasionally more than the stated volume of fluid may have been inserted into the balloon. If this fails, proceed as below in a step-wise fashion.
- Inject 5ml of air into the balloon port and then attempt to aspirate the balloon fluid again.
- Remove the plunger from the syringe leaving just the tip in the balloon port. Leaving this in place for an hour or so may allow an additional few millilitres of fluid to drain allowing deflation of the balloon.
- Cut the inflation port off the catheter. This removes the distal valve from the equation and will usually result in deflation of the balloon.
- If unsuccessful, pass the stiff end of a

guidewire down the inflation channel in an attempt to unblock the inflation port.
- If this fails, cut across the main catheter tubing 5cm away from where it emerges from the urethra, placing forceps on one edge of the cut end of the catheter (to avoid migration of the remnant tubing into the bladder).
- If still unsuccessful (or as an alternative to the above step), ultrasound-guided suprapubic percutaneous needle puncture of the balloon is indicated in male patients. In female patients, the catheter can be pulled downwards so that the balloon is at the bladder neck, allowing palpation of the balloon and needle puncture through the anterior vaginal wall.
- Endoscopic puncture of the balloon under general anaesthesia is another option although rarely needed.
- In all circumstances, the catheter must be thoroughly inspected following removal for any missing fragments (that would require cystoscopic removal).

Tip left inside the bladder
Breakage of the tip of the catheter is a recognised complication of long-term catheterisation[8]. It tends to occur at the proximal junction of the balloon with the catheter as a result of excessive force on the catheter (e.g. patient pulling or catching it inadvertently). If catheter removal is not witnessed, every effort should be made to find a missing tip in the patient's surroundings – to avoid unnecessary endoscopy.

Management
- Refer to urology for endoscopic removal of the retained fragment under local or general anaesthesia.

- If the patient is unable to void in the interim, insert a new urinary catheter to facilitate bladder drainage.

Suprapubic catheter problems

Urologists are frequently asked to see inpatients or patients in the emergency department whose SPCs have fallen out, or need to be replaced for any of the reasons highlighted above (blockages, debris, etc.). Replacement of a SPC requires urgent attention and can be attempted first without referral to a urologist.

Management

- Be aware that a mature SPC track will begin to close after just 1 hour without a catheter *in situ*. Replacement should therefore be prompt.
- To remove a SPC, simply deflate the balloon and withdraw the catheter. If there is difficulty in deflating the balloon, follow the steps described on page 164.
- Of note, the deflated ruffled balloon on the catheter can catch on the rectus sheath during withdrawal, felt as resistance (**Figure 7.10**). Ensure that the balloon is fully deflated, place a little Instillagel® alongside the SPC tract and gently pull again using a twisting motion.
- To replace a SPC, sterilise the skin and instill lignocaine jelly (e.g. Instillagel®)

into the opening. Pass a standard Foley catheter (typically silicone as it will be long-term) down the track and inflate the balloon. In female patients, inspect the perineum at the end of the procedure to ensure the catheter has not exited the bladder through the urethra.

- If the SPC track has closed and passage of the catheter is not possible, a urethral catheter can be sited instead as a temporary measure. If this is not possible (due to bladder neck closure or other anatomical problems), refer urgently to urology for assistance, where it may be possible to either dilate up the SPC tract or place a new SPC.

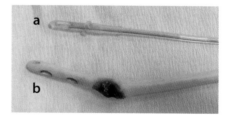

Figure 7.10 A 12 Ch 2-way silicone catheter (**a**) and a 22 Ch 3-way latex-coated catheter (**b**), both demonstrating a ruffled deflated balloon, which resulted in difficulty in a catheter removal from a patient with a reconstructed ileal bladder substitute and required general anaesthesia removal as an emergency case.

Key Points

- Many common catheter-related problems are easily managed with simple measures.
- The tips, tricks and basic management suggestions presented should enable doctors working in other specialties to appropriately manage many of these scenarios without necessarily needing to consult a specialist urology service.

LOCAL ANAESTHETIC PENILE BLOCKS[4]

The ability to obtain effective penile anaesthesia is very helpful in the management of a number of emergency urological conditions. Adequate blockade allows painless manipulation of the penis and surgical intervention involving all areas including the skin, foreskin, glans, urethra and corpora. A subcutaneous penile ring block is a particularly useful technique in the emergency setting; a formal penile block is more commonly performed by the urology team.

Indication

These techniques can be utilised to provide anaesthesia for both emergency and elective procedures (Table 7.1) as well as for symptom relief and post-operative pain management. The combination of both a short- and long-acting anaesthetic agent allows the effects to happen almost immediately and last for up to 6 hours. In patients who are unfit for general anaesthesia, operations such as circumcision can be performed with a penile block alone. A penile block is also commonly used for additional analgesia in patients undergoing penile operations under general anaesthetic.

Anatomy

Sensory penile innervation is supplied by bilateral dorsal nerves of the penis that are terminal branches of the pudendal nerve (S2–S4). They run underneath the deep fascia of the penis (Buck's fascia) at the 11 and 1 o'clock positions (**Figure 7.11**). They run lateral to the dorsal penile arteries along the shaft and eventually pass underneath the pubic symphysis, deviating laterally under each inferior pubic ramus.

Technique

This would more commonly be performed in patients in the operating theatre. With the patient appropriately consented and positioned, the genital area should be cleaned with antiseptic solution, and sterile drapes used. Check the local anaesthetic (LA) vials to ensure you have the correct solution, that it is in date, and that it does NOT contain adrenaline (which is contraindicated for use in the penis), and draw up into a syringe. The LA can be injected using a blue (23 gauge) or green (21 gauge) needle. The arch of the pubic symphysis should be palpated (**Figure 7.12**) and the needle inserted perpendicularly and advanced in a direction towards the underneath of the pubic arch at the base of the penile shaft (**Figure 7.13**). At that stage, the needle should be gently withdrawn

Table 7.1 Clinical scenarios where a local anaesthetic penile block is useful.

Emergency	Elective
Penile laceration	Circumcision
Reduction of paraphimosis	Penile biopsy
Dorsal slit/circumcision (emergency)	Frenuloplasty
Priapism	Preputioplasty
Penile fracture	Nesbitt's procedure

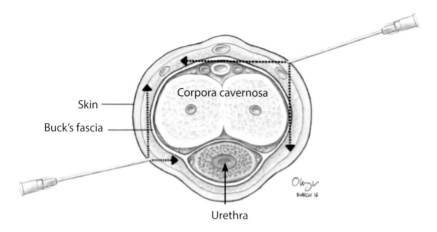

Skin

Buck's fascia

Corpora cavernosa

Urethra

Figure 7.11 Axial section of the penis, demonstrating the anatomy of the dorsal neurovascular bundle under the Buck's fascia. The dorsal penile vein is located centrally above the corpora (blue). Moving out laterally are the arteries (red) and the nerves (yellow). The technique of penile ring block is also depicted, demonstrating possible injection sites for circumferential infiltration of local anaesthetic.

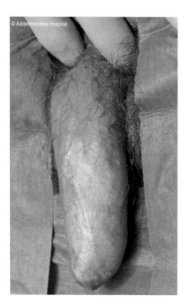

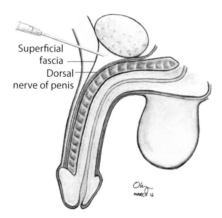

Superficial fascia
Dorsal nerve of penis

Figure 7.13 Sagittal view of the penis demonstrating the initial approach and positioning of the needle for administration of a penile block.

Figure 7.12 Palpation under the arch of the pubic symphysis.

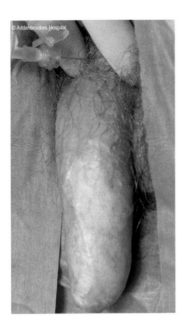

Figure 7.14 The needle is aimed to the left side underneath the inferior pubic ramus.

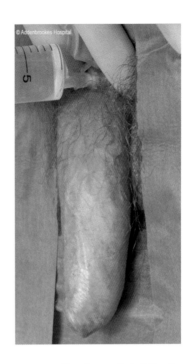

Figure 7.15 After the needle is fully advanced, aspirate to ensure the needle is not penetrating a blood vessel, and then slowly withdraw injecting 7–8ml of anaesthetic.

and angled below and to one side of the pubic symphysis aiming beneath the inferior pubic ramus (**Figure 7.14**), inserting the full length of the needle. The aim is to reach (and penetrate under) the deep penile fascia (Buck's fascia), first infiltrating down one side of the penis and then the other. Before injecting LA, aspirate to ensure you are not in a blood vessel, and if in theatre inform the anaesthetist of your intention, as inadvertent intravascular LA injection can cause arrhythmias. The needle should then be withdrawn slowly and continuously while 7–8ml of the anaesthetic agent is injected (**Figure 7.15**). The needle can either be angled towards the opposite side just under the skin surface to prevent the need for a second skin passage, or removed and a second injection performed on the other side of the penile shaft. Placing pressure at the injection site with a gauze swab will prevent formation of a haematoma. Avoid injection in the midline (12 o'clock position) to prevent penetration and direct injection of the anaesthetic into the dorsal penile vessels.

A penile block might not achieve global anaesthesia in all cases, especially for the frenular area that lies on the ventral or undersurface of the glans penis. It is helpful to combine with a partial ring block by injecting another 4–5ml of local anaesthetic at the ventral aspect of the base of the penis (**Figure 7.16**). Injection should be made in the midline (at 6 o'clock) of the underside of the penis and directed to either side respectively, creating a small bleb under the skin. Be careful not to angle too steeply, or inject too deeply, as this is where the urethra runs close to the skin.

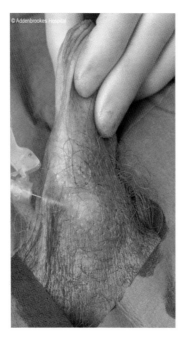

Figure 7.16 Completion of a penile block with subcutaneous injection of local anaesthetic at the ventral aspect of the base of the penis. Be careful not to penetrate too deeply, as this is where the urethra runs.

The authors use a combination of 10ml of lignocaine 1% and 10ml of chirocaine 0.5% for an adult patient in theatre. In the emergency setting, we commonly would use a smaller volume of LA (10ml 1% lignocaine) for more minor procedures (such as reduction of paraphimosis). Again, it is important not to use any adrenaline to prevent the risk of vasoconstriction leading to penile ischaemia.

Subcutaneous penile ring block

Another useful and simpler technique is a penile ring block, which may be used particularly effectively for the reduction of paraphimosis and suturing of penile lacerations. Use a small needle (23 gauge blue) and insert it superficially under the penile skin. Generally, two injection sites are required to ensure infiltration of LA circumferentially around the base of the penis (see **Figure 7.11**). The needle is advanced superficially under the skin and superficial Dartos fascia, but not as deep as the Buck's fascia. After aspiration (to exclude vessel perforation), the needle is withdrawn slowly while local anaesthetic is injected. Just before removal of the needle via the skin it should be redirected to allow for further instillation of LA in a different location around the penis (**Figure 7.11**).

Complications

Penetration of the dorsal vessels during needle placement can result in haematoma within the Buck's fascia territory. If confined to the Buck's fascia, bruising will be confined to the penis only. It is uncommon that an adequately administered penile block provides insufficient blockade – ensure adequate time is allowed for the anaesthetic to work before undertaking the penile procedure. Lignocaine insensitivity is very rare. Local anaesthetic agents combined with adrenaline should never be used because of the risk of penile ischaemia.

Key Points

- LA penile blocks are an excellent method of achieving rapid and effective anaesthesia for emergency penile procedures.
- The skill may be used in both emergency and elective settings.
- A combination of short-acting and long-acting LA without adrenaline is used.
- Serious complications are uncommon.

References

1 Harrison SC, Lawrence WT, Morley R, *et al.* British Association of Urological Surgeons' suprapubic catheter practice guidelines. *BJU Int* 2011; **107**(1): 77–85.

2 Suprapubic catheter insertion. Information for patients. 2014 (Accessed 17/11/2015); Available from: http://www.baus.org. uk/_userfiles/pages/files/Patients/Leaflets/ Suprapubic14.pdf.

3 Noel J, Wong LM, Thiruchelvam N. Urology as a specialty – are we becoming a catheter service? *BJU Int* 2013; **111**: 534–6.

4 Nyman MA, Schwenk NM, Silverstein MD. Management of urinary retention: rapid versus gradual decompression and risk of complications. *Mayo Clinic Proc* 1997; **72**: 951–6.

5 Zelhof B, Campbell IM, Bradley AJ, Young JG. Upper urinary tract trauma from urethral catheterisation in spinal cord injury patients. *Br J Med Surg Urology* 2011; **4**: 269–71.

6 Ord J, Lunn D, Reynard J. Bladder management and risk of bladder stone formation in spinal cord injured patients. *J Urology* 2003; **170**: 1734–7.

7 Linsenmeyer M, Linsenmeyer TA. Accuracy of predicting bladder stones based on catheter encrustation in individuals with spinal cord injury. *J Spinal Cord Med* 2006; **29**: 402–5.

8 Daneshmand S, Youssefzadeh D, Skinner EC. Review of techniques to remove a Foley catheter when the balloon does not deflate. *Urology* 2002; **59**: 127–9.

Chapter 8

Interventional Uroradiology Procedures

Tariq Ali and Andrew Winterbottom

Interventional radiology is a subspecialty of radiology that uses minimally invasive, image-guided techniques to both diagnose and treat conditions throughout the body. Within urology, the applications and usefulness of interventional radiology has increased significantly in recent years. There are many emergency situations where radiological procedures are safer and more effective than surgical options, and indeed other situations where interventional radiology offers the only valid treatment option. For this reason it is very important that urology and radiology departments work cohesively with one another. Outlined below are some common interventional radiology procedures used in emergency urology situations. An understanding of each procedure and its potential complications will be important when making management decisions, in preparing and communicating with the patient, and when looking after the patient after any procedure.

NEPHROSTOMY

This is a minimally invasive urinary diversion procedure, whereby, under image guidance, a drainage tube is inserted percutaneously into the renal collecting system.

Indications

In the emergency setting, a nephrostomy is usually used as a temporary urinary diversion technique to relieve obstruction and to help treat acute kidney injury or systemic sepsis (*Box 8.1*). Early intervention is crucial, particularly in the setting of a single functioning kidney (including renal transplants) to prevent progression to obstructive nephropathy.

Box 8.1 Indications for nephrostomy.

- Urinary diversion in an obstructed system (stone, tumour, clot).
- Urinary diversion away from a leak or fistula.
- Treatment of sepsis in an obstructed system that is infected.
- Access for antegrade ureteric stenting.
- Access for hybrid urological procedures (percutaneous nephrolithotomy [PCNL]).

Patient preparation

As for any procedure, baseline blood tests are essential, particularly to identify any derangement in clotting that would require correction prior to starting the procedure (*Box 8.2*). Intervening in an obstructed system increases the risk of bacteraemia and therefore adequate antibiotic cover against Gram-negative organisms is essential.

Box 8.2 General requirements for interventional procedures.

- Full blood count (FBC).
- Creatinine.
- Clotting screen.
- Antibiotic cover.

Procedure

Planning the case is essential to prevent avoidable complications. Previous computed tomography (CT) images can be helpful to identify the anatomy and to demonstrate the location of the bowel in order to prevent injury during the procedure. The procedure is usually performed with the patient in a prone position but in certain cases it may be performed in the semi-prone or supine position. The nephrostomy is performed using a combination of ultrasound (US) and fluoroscopic guidance. US is used to identify the dilated target calyx within the kidney. Adjacent bowel and pleura can also be visualised in order to prevent injury. Once the calyx has been punctured, fluoroscopy is used to image the opacified collecting system. Using a standard Seldinger technique over a guidewire, the tract is dilated and a drain inserted (**Figure 8.1**). Complications associated with the procedure are summarised in *Box 8.3*.

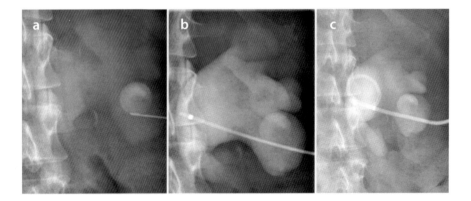

Figure 8.1 Nephrostomy insertion. Fluoroscopic images showing (**a**) initial lower pole calyx puncture; (**b**) advancement of the sheath into the renal pelvis; and (**c**) insertion of a pigtail drain into the renal pelvis.

Box 8.3 Complications of nephrostomy insertion.

- Bleeding.
- Injury to the renal tract and urine leak.
- Sepsis.
- Bowel injury.
- Pneumothorax (upper pole puncture).

Box 8.4 Indications for ureteric stenting.

- To relieve obstruction.
- To maintain ureteric patency in ureteric injuries or leak.
- To maintain ureteric patency during stone treatment.

Outcome

Nephrostomy tubes are used not only for diversion of urine in an obstructed kidney; they also provide a means of renal access for antegrade ureteric stenting and hybrid urological procedures such as percutaneous nephrolithotomy (PCNL). In some instances a nephrostomy can provide long-term renal drainage.

ANTEGRADE URETERIC STENT INSERTION

Ureteric stenting is the process by which an indwelling endoluminal tube is inserted into the ureter to ensure drainage of urine to the urinary bladder.

Indications

The indications for antegrade ureteric stenting generally follow the usual causes for obstruction of any tubular viscus, i.e. luminal causes (e.g. stone, tumour, clot), mural pathology (e.g. inflammation, tumour) or extrinsic compression (e.g. tumour, collection, fibrosis) (Box 8.4). The stent used is the same whether inserted antegrade using US and fluoroscopy or retrograde via cystoscopy.

Patient preparation

As for any procedure, baseline blood tests are essential, particularly to identify any derangement in clotting that would require correction prior to starting the procedure (Box 8.2). Intervening in an obstructed system increases the risk of bacteraemia and therefore adequate antibiotic cover against Gram-negative organisms is essential.

Procedure

Planning the case is essential to prevent avoidable complications. A CT scan is usually used to make a diagnosis, to demonstrate the level of obstruction and to identify relevant anatomy (adjacent bowel and lung). The procedure is usually performed with the patient in a prone position but in certain cases it may be performed in the semi-prone or supine position, particularly if there is pre-existing nephrostomy access. Ureteric stenting may be performed as a primary procedure or as an adjunct to an existing nephrostomy. Following renal access, a guidewire and catheter are used to negotiate the obstruction/stenosis and gain access into the urinary bladder (or conduit). The stent is then advanced over a stiff guidewire into the urinary bladder, followed by careful withdrawal of the wire and the use of a pusher/suture system to ensure a pig-tail forms both within the bladder and the renal pelvis (**Figure 8.2**). Complications associated with the procedure are summarised in *Box 8.5*.

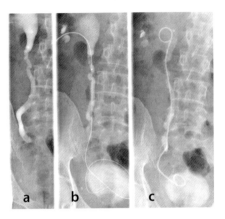

Figure 8.2 Ureteric stent. Fluoroscopic images showing (**a**) lower pole renal access with an antegrade ureterogram showing distal ureteric obstruction; (**b**) a wire has been manipulated across the ureteric obstruction into the bladder; (**c**) a ureteric stent with pigtails positioned in the renal pelvis and bladder.

Box 8.5 Complications associated with ureteric stenting.

- Bleeding.
- Injury to the renal tract and urine leak.
- Sepsis.
- Bladder irritation/stent symptoms.

Outcome

Temporary stents are usually removed cystoscopically. Long-term stents require frequent replacements to ensure patency, performed cystoscopically.

ILEAL CONDUIT ACCESS AND URETERIC STENTING

This procedure is an effective method to access the kidney via the ileal conduit in patients following ileal conduit formation often post-cystectomy.

Indications

The indications for stenting generally follow the usual causes for obstruction of any tubular viscus, i.e. luminal causes (e.g. stone, tumour, clot), mural pathology (e.g. inflammation, tumour) or extrinsic compression (e.g. tumour, collection, fibrosis) (*Box 8.6*). Common indications for intervention also include early post-operative ureteroileal leak or ischaemic stricture.

Box 8.6 Indications for ileal conduit access and ureteric stenting.

- Post-operative ureteric leak.
- Recurrent urinary tract infections (UTIs).
- Ureteric stricture (ischaemia, disease recurrence, post-operative).
- Ureteric fistula.
- Stent migration/dislodgement.

Patient preparation

Baseline blood tests are essential, particularly if an antegrade puncture is required to gain access into the ureter (*Box 8.2*). Adequate antibiotic cover against Gram-negative organisms is essential as gut flora from the conduit will reflux into the upper tracts.

Procedure

Understanding the operative anatomy is essential to identifying the position of the ureteroileal anastomosis. The procedure is usually performed retrogradely whereby a guidewire and catheter are used, via the conduit, to negotiate the ureteroileal anastomosis and gain access to the kidney. A suitable locking pigtail catheter is advanced over the wire with the pigtail positioned in the renal pelvis and the drainage port located in the stoma bag. This allows access for flushing and further imaging if required.

In some cases, retrograde access into the ureter is not possible, in which case a two-step approach is utilised. The pelvicalyceal system is accessed by direct puncture, similar to a nephrostomy, and a wire is passed down the ureter and through the stoma distally. The stoma end of the wire is then used as an access wire for the stent to be advanced retrogradely from the stoma into the pelvis of the kidney. The final position is confirmed with the injection of a small amount of contrast into the stent. If required, the direct access into the kidney may be converted into a nephrostomy (**Figure 8.3**).

Complications associated with the procedure are summarised in *Box 8.7*.

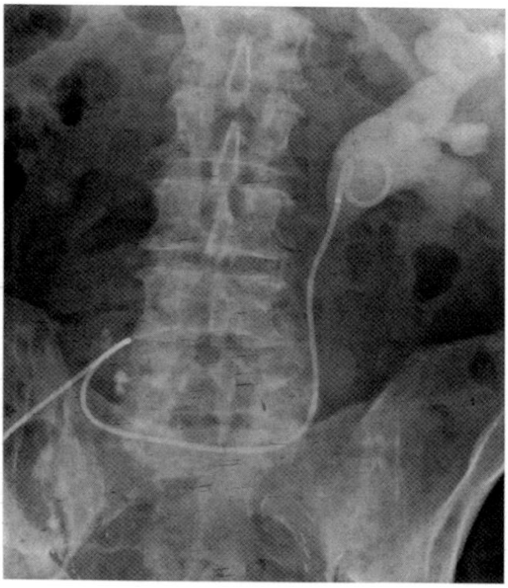

Outcome

Temporary stents are usually removed; however, in certain cases the stent is left *in situ* for a longer period of time. Indwelling stents require frequent replacements to ensure patency.

Figure 8.3 Anteroposterior fluoroscopic image showing a pigtail catheter placed retrogradely from an ileal conduit up into the left renal pelvis, which is outlined with contrast medium.

Box 8.7 Potential complications of attempted ileal conduit fluoroscopic access.

- Bleeding.
- Injury to the renal tract and urine leak.
- Sepsis.
- Conduit injury.

MITROFANOFF IMAGING/ ACCESS

This procedure is used to diagnose complications of Mitrofanoff catheterisation and establish drainage if patient self-catheterisation is not possible.

Indications

The indications for regaining access are lost access or an inability to access the Mitrofanoff, which can result in an obstructed system. An important cause for inability to self-catheterise is stricture, which may require surgical correction if recurrent.

Patient preparation

No specific preparation is required for this procedure unless there is a UTI when pre-procedure antibiotics are required. The procedure is usually performed with the patient supine.

Procedure

Initial imaging can be performed by injecting contrast medium directly into the Mitrofanoff. However, if there is obstruction, contrast simply refluxes out of the stoma. To cannulate the Mitrofanoff, a hydrophilic guidewire with the support of a catheter is used to minimise the risk of perforation. Once access is obtained, contrast medium can be injected along the length of the Mitrofanoff. A standard Foley catheter or pigtail drain of appropriate size can then be advanced over a guidewire through the Mitrofanoff (**Figure 8.4**).

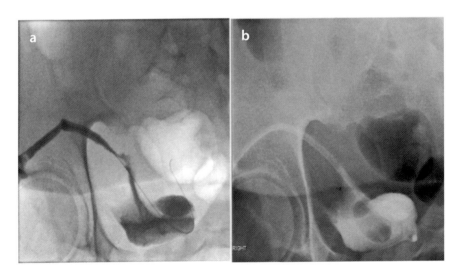

Figure 8.4 Fluoroscopic images showing (a) contrast injected retrogradely along a Mitrofanoff into the native bladder (note the guidewire already positioned in the bladder); (b) with a Foley catheter inserted with the balloon seen in the bladder.

Outcome

Complications associated with the procedure include injury to the Mitrofanoff or an inability to acquire access. If cannulation of the Mitrofanoff is not possible, then percutaneous drainage of the neobladder or native bladder can be performed.

Temporary stents are usually removed but in certain cases the stent is left *in situ* for a longer period of time. Indwelling stents require frequent replacements to ensure patency.

RENAL EMBOLISATION

This procedure involves injecting a variety of embolic material selectively into the renal arteries to occlude the target vessel.

Indications

In the emergency setting, embolisation of the renal arteries is usually performed as a minimally invasive procedure, targeting the bleeding vessel to achieve haemostasis. The commonest indications are shown in *Box 8.8*.

Patient preparation

A normal coagulation cascade is required for coils and vascular plugs to achieve haemostasis, and therefore baseline blood tests to determine clotting are required (*Box 8.9*). Antibiotic cover is not usually required. However, if large volumes of renal tissue are embolised, abscess formation is possible, so in some cases pre-procedure antibiotics should be used. Renal haemorrhage can cause a significant loss of blood volume and haemodynamic compromise to the patient. Therefore, appropriate fluid resuscitation and/or blood transfusion is vital. Constant monitoring by trained medical staff is essential to address any acute clinical deterioration. Embolisation procedures can be performed under local anaesthetic. Pain relief may be important to improve patient compliance with the procedure.

Procedure

Planning the case is essential to prevent avoidable complications, particularly 'non-target' embolisation. A triple-phase CT scan is the investigation of choice for acute renal injury of all causes. The arterial phase can

Box 8.8 Indications for renal embolisation.

- Traumatic acute renal haemorrhage (iatrogenic, blunt/penetrating injuries).
- Renal artery aneurysm/pseudoaneurysm.
- Tumour bleed (renal cell carcinoma [RCC], angiomyolipoma [AML]).

Box 8.9 Patient preparation for renal embolisation.

- FBC.
- Creatinine.
- Clotting screen.
- Close monitoring.

be used to make a reconstructed image to act as a 'roadmap' to guide therapy.

Selective embolisation is usually recommended to preserve renal function; however, in significant renal injury with large volumes of blood loss, it may be necessary to sacrifice the whole kidney by embolising the main renal artery.

Embolic agents

Several embolic agents are available and anatomy will determine the embolic agent selected in each case. Whichever material is used the basic principle is to embolise as close to the bleeding artery as possible in order to prevent 'non-target' embolisation and preserve renal function.

Access is usually via a femoral artery puncture. A selective renal artery angiogram demonstrates the site of active bleeding or pseudoaneurysm that corresponds with the reformatted images acquired from the CT scan. The catheter is advanced to the site of bleeding and embolic material delivered. An example of a clinical case is demonstrated in **Figure 8.5**. A patient presents with a penetrating knife wound to the kidney (**a**), followed by renal bleeding from the renal laceration after the blade

is removed (**b**). **Figure 8.5c** demonstrates renal bleeding on angiography that stops after embolisation, and **Figure 8.5d** demonstrates pre- and post-renal embolisation appearances on CT scan.

Complications associated with the procedure are summarised in *Box 8.10*.

Outcome

Once haemostasis is achieved, the patient is monitored and generally no further intervention is required. Close monitoring is essential to identify evidence of further bleeding.

Box 8.10 Potential complications from renal embolisation.

- Non-target embolisation.
- Renal impairment.
- Post-embolisation syndrome (low-grade fever, body aches, lethargy).
- Infection/abscess formation.
- Renal artery dissection.
- Failed embolisation.

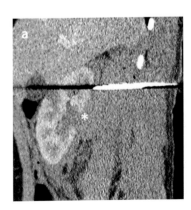

Figure 8.5 (a) Sagittal computed tomography (CT) image showing a knife blade adjacent to the upper pole of the right kidney with cortical laceration and an adjacent haematoma (asterisk);
Figure continued overleaf.

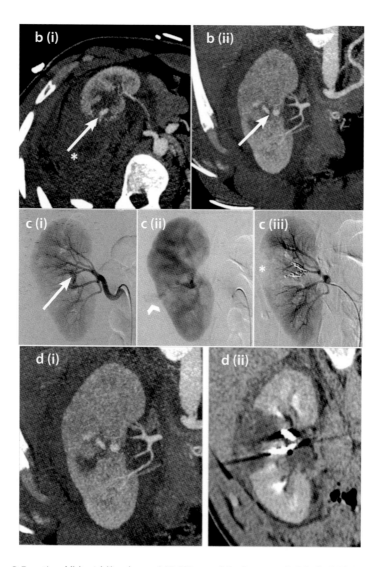

Figure 8.5 *continued* (**b**) axial (i) and coronal (ii) CT images following removal of the knife blade with active bleeding from the renal laceration (arrow) into the adjacent haematoma (asterisk); (**c**) digital subtraction angiograms showing active bleeding at the renal hilum in the arterial phase (i), bleeding into the perinephric haematoma in the later cortical phase (broad white arrow in ii) and (iii) no bleeding following coil embolisation with only a small region of reduced cortical perfusion (asterisk); (**d**) coronal CT images (i) pre-embolisation showing the initial active bleeding at the renal hilum and (ii) post-embolisation showing the embolisation coils with an adjacent localised region of cortical interpolar infarct but preservation of perfusion to both upper and lower poles.

DRAINAGE OF COLLECTIONS

Indications

Common causes of collections relevant to emergency urology include a urinoma due to renal tract trauma or post-operative leak, post-operative lymphocoele and renal abscess (*Box 8.11*).

Patient preparation

As for any interventional procedure, baseline blood tests are essential, particularly to identify any derangements in clotting that would require correction prior to starting the procedure (*Box 8.2*). There is an increased risk of bacteraemia when intervening in an infected collection and therefore adequate antibiotic cover is essential.

Procedure

Planning the case is essential to prevent avoidable complications. A review of previous imaging is essential to identify the site of the collection and plan drainage. Depending on the location and operator preference, both CT and US can be used to guide the drainage procedure. As with most radiologically-guided drainage procedures, a standard Seldinger technique is used to insert a pigtail drainage catheter into the collection.

Complications associated with the procedure are summarised in *Box 8.12*.

Outcome

The drained fluid should be sent for microbiological assessment in cases of sepsis and can also be sent for biochemistry assessment to differentiate a urinoma from a lymphocoele. Once the collection has been adequately drained, then the drain can be removed. This is generally guided by improvement in patient symptoms and reducing drain output.

Box 8.11 Indications for radiological drainage of collections in urology.

- Urinoma (trauma).
- Lymphocoele.
- Abscess.

Box 8.12 Potential complications of drain insertion.

- Bleeding.
- Injury to surrounding structures.
- Sepsis.

Key Points

- Baseline bloods, including a coagulation screen, should be available before requesting interventional procedures.
- Antibiotic cover should be given for any procedures involving infected or static urine.
- A cohesive relationship between urology and interventional radiology is crucial.

References

1 Alago W Jr, Sofocleous CT, Covey AM, *et al*. Placement of transileal conduit retrograde nephroureteral stents in patients with ureteral obstruction after cystectomy: technique and outcome. *Am J Roentgenol* 2008; **191**: 1536–9.

2 Dyer RB, Regan JD, Kavanagh PV, *et al*. Percutaneous nephrostomy with extensions of the technique: step by step. *Radiographics* 2002; **22**(3): 503–25.

3 Kessel D, Robertson I. *Interventional Radiology. A Survival Guide*, 3rd edn. Churchill Livingstone Elsevier, London, 2010.

4 Makramalla A, Zuckerman DA. Nephroureteral stents: principles and techniques. *Semin Intervent Radiol* 2011; **28**: 367–79.

5 Poulakis V, Ferakis N, Becht E, *et al*. Treatment of renal-vascular injury by transcatheter embolization: immediate and long-term effects on renal function. *J Endourol* 2006; **20**: 405–9.

EXAMPLE EMERGENCY DEPARTMENT PROTOCOL FOR SUSPECTED SEPSIS

Reproduced with the kind permission of the UK Sepsis Trust. http://www.sepsistrust.org/.

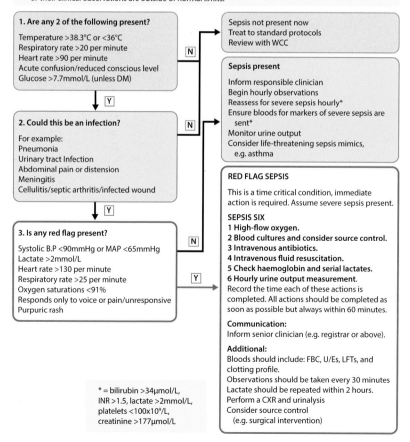

Sepsis is a time critical condition. Screening, early intervention and immediate treatment saves lives. This tool should be applied to all adult patients who are not pregnant who have a suspected infection or their clinical observations are outside of normal limits.

1. Are any 2 of the following present?

Temperature >38.3°C or <36°C
Respiratory rate >20 per minute
Heart rate >90 per minute
Acute confusion/reduced conscious level
Glucose >7.7mmol/L (unless DM)

N → **Sepsis not present now**
Treat to standard protocols
Review with WCC

Y ↓

2. Could this be an infection?

For example:
Pneumonia
Urinary tract Infection
Abdominal pain or distension
Meningitis
Cellulitis/septic arthritis/infected wound

N → **Sepsis present**

Inform responsible clinician
Begin hourly observations
Reassess for severe sepsis hourly*
Ensure bloods for markers of severe sepsis are sent*
Monitor urine output
Consider life-threatening sepsis mimics, e.g. asthma

Y ↓

3. Is any red flag present?

Systolic B.P <90mmHg or MAP <65mmHg
Lactate >2mmol/L
Heart rate >130 per minute
Respiratory rate >25 per minute
Oxygen saturations <91%
Responds only to voice or pain/unresponsive
Purpuric rash

N →

Y →

RED FLAG SEPSIS

This is a time critical condition, immediate action is required. Assume severe sepsis present.

SEPSIS SIX
1 High-flow oxygen.
2 Blood cultures and consider source control.
3 Intravenous antibiotics.
4 Intravenous fluid resuscitation.
5 Check haemoglobin and serial lactates.
6 Hourly urine output measurement.
Record the time each of these actions is completed. All actions should be completed as soon as possible but always within 60 minutes.

Communication:
Inform senior clinician (e.g. registrar or above).

Additional:
Bloods should include: FBC, U/Es, LFTs, and clotting profile.
Observations should be taken every 30 minutes
Lactate should be repeated within 2 hours.
Perform a CXR and urinalysis
Consider source control
  (e.g. surgical intervention)

* = bilirubin >34μmol/L, INR >1.5, lactate >2mmol/L, platelets <100x10⁹/L, creatinine >177μmol/L

THE ABCDE APPROACH

Reproduced with the kind permission of the Resuscitation Council (UK).

Underlying principles

The approach to all deteriorating or critically ill patients is the same. The underlying principles are:

- Use the Airway, Breathing, Circulation, Disability, Exposure (ABCDE) approach to assess and treat the patient.
- Do a complete initial assessment and reassess regularly.
- Treat life-threatening problems before moving to the next part of the assessment.
- Assess the effects of treatment.
- Recognise when you will need extra help. Call for appropriate help early.
- Use all members of the team. This enables interventions (e.g. assessment, attaching monitors, intravenous [IV] access), to be undertaken simultaneously.
- Communicate effectively – use the Situation, Background, Assessment, Recommendation (SBAR) or Reason, Story, Vital signs, Plan (RSVP) approach.
- The aim of the initial treatment is to keep the patient alive, and achieve some clinical improvement. This will buy time for further treatment and making a diagnosis.

- Remember, it can take a few minutes for treatments to work, so wait a short while before reassessing the patient after an intervention.

First steps

- Ensure personal safety. Wear an apron and gloves as appropriate.
- First look at the patient in general to see if the patient appears unwell.
- If the patient is awake, ask "How are you?". If the patient appears unconscious or has collapsed, shake him and ask "Are you alright?" If he responds normally he has a patent airway, is breathing and has brain perfusion. If he speaks only in short sentences, he may have breathing problems. Failure of the patient to respond is a clear marker of critical illness.
- This first rapid 'Look, Listen and Feel' of the patient should take about 30 seconds and will often indicate a patient is critically ill and there is a need for urgent help. Ask a colleague to ensure appropriate help is coming.
- If the patient is unconscious, unresponsive, and is not breathing

normally (occasional gasps are not normal), start cardiopulmonary resuscitation (CPR) according to the resuscitation guidelines. If you are confident and trained to do so, feel for a pulse to determine if the patient has a respiratory arrest. If there are any doubts about the presence of a pulse start CPR.

- Monitor the vital signs early. Attach a pulse oximeter, electrocardiogram (ECG) monitor and a non-invasive blood pressure (BP) monitor to all critically ill patients, as soon as possible.
- Insert an IV cannula as soon as possible. Take bloods for investigation when inserting the IV cannula.

Airway (A)

Airway obstruction is an emergency. Get expert help immediately. Untreated, airway obstruction causes hypoxia and risks damage to the brain, kidneys and heart, cardiac arrest and death.

- Look for the signs of airway obstruction:
  › Airway obstruction causes paradoxical chest and abdominal movements ('see-saw' respirations) and the use of the accessory muscles of respiration. Central cyanosis is a late sign of airway obstruction. In complete airway obstruction, there are no breath sounds at the mouth or nose. In partial obstruction, air entry is diminished and often noisy.
  › In the critically ill patient, depressed consciousness often leads to airway obstruction.
- Treat airway obstruction as a medical emergency:

  › Obtain expert help immediately. Untreated, airway obstruction causes hypoxaemia (low PaO_2) with the risk of hypoxic injury to the brain, kidneys and heart, cardiac arrest and even death.
  › In most cases, only simple methods of airway clearance are required (e.g. airway opening manoeuvres, airways suction, insertion of an oropharyngeal or nasopharyngeal airway). Tracheal intubation may be required when these fail.
- Give oxygen at high concentration:
  › Provide high-concentration oxygen using a mask with oxygen reservoir. Ensure that the oxygen flow is sufficient (usually 15L/min) to prevent collapse of the reservoir during inspiration. If the patient's trachea is intubated, give high-concentration oxygen with a self-inflating bag.
  › In acute respiratory failure, aim to maintain an oxygen saturation of 94–98%. In patients at risk of hypercapnic respiratory failure (see below), aim for an oxygen saturation of 88–92%.

Breathing (B)

During the immediate assessment of breathing, it is vital to diagnose and treat immediately life-threatening conditions (e.g. acute severe asthma, pulmonary oedema, tension pneumothorax and massive haemothorax).

- Look, listen and feel for the general signs of respiratory distress: sweating, central cyanosis, use of the accessory muscles of respiration, and abdominal breathing.

- Count the respiratory rate. The normal rate is 12–20 breaths/min. A high (>25/min) or increasing respiratory rate is a marker of illness and a warning that the patient may deteriorate suddenly.
- Assess the depth of each breath, the pattern (rhythm) of respiration and whether chest expansion is equal on both sides.
- Note any chest deformity (this may increase the risk of deterioration in the ability to breathe normally); look for a raised jugular venous pulse (JVP) (e.g. in acute severe asthma or a tension pneumothorax); note the presence and patency of any chest drains; remember that abdominal distension may limit diaphragmatic movement, thereby worsening respiratory distress.
- Record the inspired oxygen concentration (%) and the SpO_2 reading of the pulse oximeter. The pulse oximeter does not detect hypercapnia. If the patient is receiving supplemental oxygen, the SpO_2 may be normal in the presence of a very high $PaCO_2$.
- Listen to the patient's breath sounds a short distance from his face: rattling airway noises indicate the presence of airway secretions, usually caused by the inability of the patient to cough sufficiently or to take a deep breath. Stridor or wheeze suggests partial, but significant, airway obstruction.
- Percuss the chest: hyperresonance may suggest a pneumothorax; dullness usually indicates consolidation or pleural fluid.
- Auscultate the chest: bronchial breathing indicates lung consolidation with patent airways; absent or reduced sounds suggest a pneumothorax or pleural fluid or lung consolidation caused by complete obstruction.
- Check the position of the trachea in the suprasternal notch: deviation to one side indicates mediastinal shift (e.g. pneumothorax, lung fibrosis or pleural fluid).
- Feel the chest wall to detect surgical emphysema or crepitus (suggesting a pneumothorax until proven otherwise).
- The specific treatment of respiratory disorders depends upon the cause. Nevertheless, all critically ill patients should be given oxygen. In a subgroup of patients with chronic obstructive pulmonary disease (COPD), high concentrations of oxygen may depress breathing (i.e. they are at risk of hypercapnic respiratory failure, often referred to as type 2 respiratory failure). Nevertheless, these patients will also sustain end-organ damage or cardiac arrest if their blood oxygen tensions are allowed to decrease. In this group, aim for a lower than normal PaO_2 and oxygen saturation. Give oxygen via a Venturi 28% mask (4L/min) or a 24% Venturi mask (4L/min) initially and reassess. Aim for a target SpO_2 range of 88–92% in most COPD patients, but evaluate the target for each patient based on the patient's arterial blood gas measurements during previous exacerbations (if available). Some patients with chronic lung disease carry an oxygen alert card (that documents their target saturation) and their own appropriate Venturi mask.
- If the patient's depth or rate of breathing is judged to be inadequate, or absent, use a bag-mask or pocket mask ventilation to improve oxygenation and ventilation, whilst

calling immediately for expert help. In cooperative patients who do not have airway obstruction, consider the use of non-invasive ventilation (NIV). In patients with an acute exacerbation of COPD, the use of NIV is often helpful and prevents the need for tracheal intubation and invasive ventilation.

Circulation (C)

In almost all medical and surgical emergencies, consider hypovolaemia to be the primary cause of shock, until proven otherwise. Unless there are obvious signs of a cardiac cause, give IV fluid to any patient with cool peripheries and a fast heart rate. In surgical patients, rapidly exclude haemorrhage (overt or hidden). Remember that breathing problems, such as a tension pneumothorax, can also compromise a patient's circulatory state. This should have been treated earlier on in the assessment.

- Look at the colour of the hands and digits: are they blue, pink, pale or mottled?
- Assess the limb temperature by feeling the patient's hands: are they cool or warm?
- Measure the capillary refill time (CRT). Apply cutaneous pressure for 5 seconds on a fingertip held at heart level (or just above) with enough pressure to cause blanching. Time how long it takes for the skin to return to the colour of the surrounding skin after releasing the pressure. The normal value for CRT is usually <2 seconds. A prolonged CRT suggests poor peripheral perfusion. Other factors (e.g. cold surroundings, poor lighting, old age) can prolong CRT.
- Assess the state of the veins: they may be underfilled or collapsed when hypovolaemia is present.
- Count the patient's pulse rate (or preferably heart rate by listening to the heart with a stethoscope).
- Palpate peripheral and central pulses, assessing for presence, rate, quality, regularity and equality. Barely palpable central pulses suggest a poor cardiac output, whilst a bounding pulse may indicate sepsis.
- Measure the patient's BP. Even in shock, the BP may be normal, because compensatory mechanisms increase peripheral resistance in response to reduced cardiac output. A low diastolic BP suggests arterial vasodilation (as in anaphylaxis or sepsis). A narrowed pulse pressure (difference between systolic and diastolic pressures; normally 35–45mmHg) suggests arterial vasoconstriction (cardiogenic shock or hypovolaemia) and may occur with rapid tachyarrhythmia.
- Auscultate the heart. Is there a murmur or pericardial rub? Are the heart sounds difficult to hear? Does the audible heart rate correspond to the pulse rate?
- Look for other signs of poor cardiac output, such as a reduced conscious level and, if the patient has a urinary catheter, oliguria (urine volume <0.5ml/kg/h).
- Look thoroughly for external haemorrhage from wounds or drains or evidence of concealed haemorrhage (e.g. thoracic, intraperitoneal, retroperitoneal or into the gut). Intrathoracic, intra-abdominal or pelvic blood loss may be significant, even if drains are empty.
- The specific treatment of cardiovascular collapse depends on the cause,

but should be directed at fluid replacement, haemorrhage control and restoration of tissue perfusion. Seek the signs of conditions that are immediately life-threatening (e.g. cardiac tamponade, massive or continuing haemorrhage, septicaemic shock), and treat them urgently.

- Insert one or more large (14 or 16 G) IV cannulae. Use short, wide-bore cannulae, because they enable the highest flow.
- Take blood from the cannula for routine haematological, biochemical, coagulation and microbiological investigations and cross-matching, before infusing IV fluid.
- Give a bolus of 500ml of warmed crystalloid solution (e.g. Hartmann's solution or 0.9% sodium chloride) over less than 15 minutes if the patient is hypotensive. Use smaller volumes (e.g. 250ml) for patients with known cardiac failure or trauma and use closer monitoring (listen to the chest for crackles after each bolus).
- Reassess the heart rate and BP regularly (every 5 minutes), aiming for the patient's normal BP or, if this is unknown, a target >100mmHg systolic.
- If the patient does not improve, repeat the fluid challenge. Seek expert help if there is a lack of response to repeated fluid boluses.
- If symptoms and signs of cardiac failure (dyspnoea, increased heart rate, raised JVP, a third heart sound and pulmonary crackles on auscultation) occur, decrease the fluid infusion rate or stop the fluids altogether. Seek alternative means of improving tissue perfusion (e.g. inotropes or vasopressors).
- If the patient has primary chest pain and

a suspected acute coronary syndrome (ACS), record a 12-lead ECG early.
- Immediate general treatment for ACS includes:
  › Aspirin 300mg, orally, crushed or chewed, as soon as possible.
  › Nitroglycerine, as sublingual glyceryl trinitrate (tablet or spray).
  › Oxygen: only give oxygen if the patient's SpO_2 is less than 94% breathing air alone.
  › Morphine (or diamorphine) titrated IV to avoid sedation and respiratory depression.

Disability (D)

- Common causes of unconsciousness include profound hypoxia, hypercapnia, cerebral hypoperfusion, or the recent administration of sedatives or analgesic drugs.
- Review and treat the ABCs: exclude or treat hypoxia and hypotension.
- Check the patient's drug chart for reversible drug-induced causes of depressed consciousness. Give an antagonist where appropriate (e.g. naloxone for opioid toxicity).
- Examine the pupils (size, equality and reaction to light).
- Make a rapid initial assessment of the patient's conscious level using the AVPU method: Alert, responds to Vocal stimuli, responds to Painful stimuli or Unresponsive to all stimuli. Alternatively, use the Glasgow Coma Scale score. A painful stimuli can be given by applying supra-orbital pressure (at the supra-orbital notch).
- Measure the blood glucose to exclude hypoglycaemia using a rapid finger-prick bedside testing method. In a peri-arrest patient use a venous or arterial

blood sample for glucose measurement as fingerprick sample glucose measurements can be unreliable in sick patients. Follow local protocols for the management of hypoglycaemia. For example, if the blood sugar is less than 4.0mmol/L in an unconscious patient, give an initial dose of 50ml of 10% glucose solution IV. If necessary, give further doses of IV 10% glucose every minute until the patient has fully regained consciousness, or a total of 250ml of 10% glucose has been given. Repeat blood glucose measurements to monitor the effects of treatment. If there is no improvement consider further doses of 10% glucose. Specific national guidance exists for the management of hypoglycaemia in adults with diabetes mellitus.
- Nurse unconscious patients in the lateral position if their airway is not protected.

Exposure (E)
- To examine the patient properly full exposure of the body may be necessary. Respect the patient's dignity and minimise heat loss.

Additional information
- Take a full clinical history from the patient, any relatives or friends, and other staff.
- Review the patient's notes and charts:
  › Study both absolute and trended values of vital signs.
  › Check that important routine medications are prescribed and being given.
- Review the results of laboratory or radiological investigations.
- Consider which level of care is required by the patient (e.g. ward, high-dependency unit, intensive care unit).
- Make complete entries in the patient's notes of your findings, assessment and treatment. Where necessary, hand over the patient to your colleagues.
- Record the patient's response to therapy.
- Consider definitive treatment of the patient's underlying condition.

Index